Foundations of Chinese Medicine

Foundations of Chinese Medicine

Penny Welsh

STATES
ACADEMIC PRESS
www.statesacademicpress.com

States Academic Press,
109 South 5th Street,
Brooklyn, NY 11249, USA

Visit us on the World Wide Web at:
www.statesacademicpress.com

ISBN: 978-1-63989-214-3 (Hardback)

Cataloging-in-Publication Data

Foundations of Chinese medicine / Penny Welsh.
p. cm.
Includes bibliographical references and index.
ISBN 978-1-63989-214-3
1. Medicine, Chinese. 2. Alternative medicine. 3. Medicine. I. Welsh, Penny.
R601 .F68 2022
610.951--dc23

TABLE OF CONTENTS

PREFACE

This book is a culmination of my many years of practice in this field. I attribute the success of this book to my support group. I would like to thank my parents who have showered me with unconditional love and support and my peers and professors for their constant guidance.

Chinese medicine is a sub-field of traditional medicine. It involves the usage of various forms of acupuncture, gua sha, herbal medicine, cupping therapy and dietary therapy. The basic principle of this field is that body's vital energy is moving through channels known as meridians and that it is connected to bodily organs and functions through branches. The basis of this field is rooted in the cosmological notions like five phases and yin-yang. According to this discipline, health is the interaction of internal and external entities and that disease arises because of disharmony. It is concerned primarily with the body's functions like breathing, digestion and temperature maintenance. This book is a valuable compilation of topics, ranging from the basic to the most complex theories and principles related to this field. It also unfolds the innovative aspects of chinese medicine which will be crucial for the holistic understanding of the subject matter. In this book, constant effort has been made to make the understanding of the difficult concepts of this discipline as easy and informative as possible, for the readers.

The details of chapters are provided below for a progressive learning:

Chapter - Introduction

Traditional Chinese medicine is a branch of traditional medicine which is based on Chinese medical practices that includes various forms of herbal medicines and therapies such as acupuncture, cupping therapy, massage and dietary therapy. The most widely used substance for most of the cures is Ginseng. This is an introductory chapter which will briefly introduce all the types of medicines and therapies used in traditional Chinese medicine.

Chapter - The Body in Traditional Chinese Medicine

Traditional Chinese medicine believes in the circulation of the body's vital energy through channels known as meridians that are connected to body organs and functions. It divides the body into five fundamental substances - Qi, Xue, Jin ye, Zang-fu and Jing Luo. The chapter closely examines the model of body in traditional Chinese medicine to provide an extensive understanding of the subject.

Chapter - The Theory of Yin and Yang

Yin and Yang is a theory that describes how the opposite forces are interconnected, complementary and interdependent in the natural world. It divides the body organs into Yin and Yang. Yin organs include liver, heart, spleen, lung and kidney, while Yang organs are gall bladder, small intestine, stomach, large intestine, triple burner and urinary bladder. This chapter has been carefully written to provide an easy understanding of the theory of Yin and Yang.

Chapter – The Five Elements

Wu Xing are the five types of energies, dominating at different types. The names of the "Five Phases" are metal, wood, water, fire and earth. This chapter closely examines the elements of Wu Xing to provide an extensive understanding of the subject.

Chapter – The Concept of Illness

In traditional Chinese medicine, illness is an imbalance of qi and Yin-Yang rather than a purely physical phenomenon. It follows eight principles of diagnosis that are Yin and Yang, interior, exterior, heat, cold, deficiency and excess. The topics elaborated in this chapter will help in gaining a better perspective about the related concepts of illness and diagnosis in traditional Chinese medicine.

Chapter – Chinese Therapies

The Chinese therapies are used for improving sleep quality, balancing hormones, reducing side effects of chemotherapy and radiation, treating neuropathy, stress, arthritis, etc. Some of the most common therapies are cupping, Gua sha, Tui na, Qigong, and Chinese food therapy. This chapter closely examines these therapies of traditional Chinese medicine to provide an extensive understanding of the subject.

Chapter – Chinese Herbal Medicine

Chinese herbal medicine includes various remedies, herbs, therapies such as Chinese herbal therapy, Chinese patent medicine, tonifying herbs, downward draining herbs, etc. The topics elaborated in this chapter will help in gaining a better perspective of the aspects related to Chinese herbal medicine.

Chapter – Acupuncture, Acupressure and Moxibustion

Acupuncture refers to the practice of inserting needles into the body for reducing pain and boosting well-being and curing some illnesses. Acupressure is the application of pressure to acupuncture points on a body for the relief of tension and pain. Moxibustion is a Chinese medicine therapy in which dried mugwort is burned on particular points on the body for various therapeutic effects. This chapter discusses acupuncture, acupressure and moxibustion in detail.

Penny Welsh

Introduction

CHAPTER 1

Traditional Chinese medicine is a branch of traditional medicine which is based on Chinese medical practices that includes various forms of herbal medicines and therapies such as acupuncture, cupping therapy, massage and dietary therapy. The most widely used substance for most of the cures is Ginseng. This is an introductory chapter which will briefly introduce all the types of medicines and therapies used in traditional Chinese medicine.

TRADITIONAL CHINESE MEDICINE

Traditional Chinese Medicine, is a profound pathway to create the life you truly want to live, the life you were born to live. It's a timeless bridge that can initiate and support change and growth in any and every life dimension: physical, mental, emotional, and spiritual.

TCM has the power to unlock your true potential and help you develop and use your own unique gifts and talents. Its insightful wisdom and ability to understand and address individual health needs empowers each person with a way to unite body, mind, and spirit—the foundation for lasting, authentic health. TCM teaches you how to live a life of balance, wellness, and harmony.

It's true that TCM is one of the oldest healing systems on the planet. It has actually been in continuous practice for thousands of years. How can something so old still work for people living today—in your life?

TCM can be effectively applied to help heal anyone and any health issue no matter what year it is because it's rooted in unchanging natural law, which has its source beyond time. This unique paradigm of medicine grew out of penetrating observation of how everything in our reality functions at the deepest, invisible levels and interacts with the surface or visible physical levels. It's a medicine of extraordinary relationships. Every TCM principle, theory, and healing practice reflects and harmonizes with the relationships that exist within natural law.

Four Key TCM Principles

- Your body is an integrated whole: Each and every structure in your body is an integral and necessary part of the whole. Along with your mind, emotions, and spirit, your physical body structures form a miraculously complex, interrelated system that is powered by life force, or energy.

- You are completely connected to nature: Changes in nature are always reflected in your body. TCM factors in the particular season, geographical location, time of day, as well as your age, genetics, and the condition of your body when looking at your health issues.
- You were born with a natural self-healing ability: Your body is a microcosm that reflects the macrocosm. Think about it: nature has a regenerative capacity, and so do you. Sometimes, this ability may appear to be lost or difficult to access. In most cases, it is never completely gone.
- Prevention is the best cure: Do you know your body is continually revealing signs about the state of your health? Let's face it, it's common to ignore these signs or symptoms until something more complicated arises. TCM teaches you how to interpret what your body is telling you.

Health Benefits

To date, Western scientists have not extensively studied the use of traditional Chinese medicine in the treatment of specific health conditions. However, traditional Chinese medicine is used to address the following conditions:

- Allergies.
- Anxiety.
- Arthritis (e.g. rheumatoid arthritis).
- Back pain.
- Depression.
- Diabetes.
- Eczema, hives, acne, psoriasis, and other skin conditions.
- Fertility.
- High blood pressure.
- Insomnia.
- Menopause symptoms.
- Obesity.
- Parkinson's disease.

Although standard treatment in modern medicine is based on the diagnosis, in TCM, the treatment would depend on the underlying imbalance. For example, a person with insomnia may have difficulty sleeping because of an imbalance such as a kidney yin deficiency, spleen qi deficiency, or blood deficiency.

Unique Approach

Rooted in a philosophy known as Taoism, traditional Chinese medicine is based on the theory that all of the body's organs mutually support each other. Therefore, in order to be healthy, an individual's organs (and their functions) must be in balance. This balance is attained, in part, by harmonizing yin and yang, two opposing but complementary energies thought to affect all life.

Another theory in traditional Chinese medicine is that vital energy (called "qi" or "chi") flows throughout the body via certain pathways (or "meridians"). According to this theory, disease and other emotional, mental, and physical health problems develop when the flow of qi is blocked, weak, or excessive. Restoring the flow of qi is considered essential to balancing the yin and yang and, in turn, achieving wellness.

What to Expect?

During a typical appointment, a TCM practitioner would assess your overall health by taking a health history, doing a tongue assessment, pulse assessment, and a physical exam. The exam would identify any Imbalances or qi blockages.

If the practitioner identifies an imbalance in one of TCM's organ systems, it doesn't necessarily mean that the person has a physical disease in that organ.

The liver, for instance, helps to regulate the smooth flow of qi. If a person has "liver qi stagnation", the energy is said to be blocked, resulting in irritability, anger, or depression, a bitter taste in the mouth, indigestion, and a pulse that practitioners describe as "wiry".

A "kidney yin deficiency", on the other hand, is associated with a dry mouth, hot flushes in the afternoon or evening, tinnitus, and forgetfulness. The tongue is usually reddish in color with little or no tongue coating. Practitioners describe the pulse as "floating".

Treatment Methods

There are many different therapeutic methods used in traditional Chinese medicine, the most popular being acupuncture. Since traditional Chinese medicine emphasizes individualized treatment, healing methods vary widely from patient to patient. These methods often include:

- Acupuncture: Though acupuncture's roots lie in TCM, it is used as a western treatment for a variety of health concerns.

- Acupressure: Finger pressure is applied over acupuncture points and meridians.

Cupping Therapy

Diet and nutrition: Foods are thought to have warming/cooling properties and are said to have specific healing properties.

- Herbal medicine: Herbs and herbal tea may be suggested.
- Moxibustion: A practice that involves burning an herb near the skin to warm the area over acupuncture points.
- Tuina: A type of bodywork that combines massage and acupressure.

  Exercises such as tai chi and qi gong.

TCM Herbs

Rather than prescribing specific herbs, practitioners of traditional Chinese medicine typically combine a number of different herbs in formulas selected depending on the patient's individual needs. These formulas may be given as teas, capsules, tinctures, or powders.

Herbs commonly used in traditional Chinese medicine include:

- Astragalus,
- Ginkgo biloba,
- Red yeast rice,
- Cinnamon,
- Ginger,
- Ginseng,
- Gotu kola.

While consumers face risks when purchasing any dietary supplement (such as contamination with other substances) due to a lack of regulation, these risks may be of greater magnitude with herbal products that have been manufactured abroad, particularly those containing a variety of herbs.

Vitamins-Minerals

Traditional Chinese medical (TCM) theory has been developed over many centuries and the core ideology pre-dates the discovery of individual vitamins and minerals which is relatively recent. However, with a modern understanding of how these substances can benefit the body it is easy to overlay them with specific TCM archetypes based on Chinese medicine with a few liberties taken. Most vitamins and mineral impact multiple organs and elements. Note: This is a theoretical exercise with the understanding that these substances would be of benefit only in the case that they are lacking.

Five Elements

Five Element theory of traditional Chinese medicine associates energetic organ systems, emotions, sensory organs, and all of the related symptoms of each element. It is a core tool of Chinese medicine to allow practitioners of Asian medicine to form an accurate diagnosis and appropriate treatment plan.

Water Element of Chinese Medicine

Vitamin A

- Benefits the ears.
- Nourishes the mucous membranes of the Urinary Bladder.

Vitamin B-7 Biotin

- Influences healthy hair growth.

Vitamin B-9 Folate

- Promotes the DNA synthesis and generates structure.
- Vital to reproduction.
- Protects Kidney Yin.

Vitamin B-12 Cobalamin

- Essential for healthy growth and the utilization of our DNA blueprint.

Vitamin C Ascorbic Acid

- Directionally rises and holds the hair.
- Treats bladder infections.
- Benefits the spine and prevents back problems.

Wood Element of Chinese Medicine

Vitamin A

- Benefits the eyes.

Vitamin B-1 Thiamine

- Allows Liver to fulfill its function of storing and thus prevents Liver Yang Rising (high blood pressure).
- Deficiency can contribute to Liver Qi Stagnation.
- Benefits the eyes.
- Combats depression and irritability.
- Associated with a lack of motivation when deficient.

Vitamin B-3 Niacin

- Associated with arthritis if deficient.

Vitamin B-6 Pyridoxine

- Associated with headaches and depression.
- Prevents Liver attacking the Spleen due to Liver Qi Congestion.
- Promotes liver's ability to break down fatty acids.
- Associated with hormonal balance in women.

Vitamin B-7 Biotin

- Promotes liver's ability to break down fatty acids.
- Used in conditions with Internal Wind (likely due to Liver Congestion-think Parkinson's disease).
- Associated with unexplained mood disorders and mood swings.

Vitamin B-9 Folate

- Used in conditions with Internal Wind (likely due to Liver Congestion-think Restless Leg Syndrome).

Vitamin C Ascorbic Acid

- Associated with treating gallstones.
- Benefits the Liver.
- Combats arthritis.

Vitamin E d-alpha Tocopherol

- Benefits the eyes (reinforces blood vessels of eye).
- Fire Element of Chinese Medicine.

Vitamin B-1 Thiamine

- Contributes to emotional health.
- Strengthens the Heart muscle.

Vitamin B-3 Niacin

- Breaks up Blood Stagnation.
- Calms the Shen (necessary for psychological balances).

Vitamin B-6 Pyridoxine

- Associated with Heart Health (clotting factors).

Vitamin B-12 Cobalamin

- Associated with psychological disorders due to neurological issues.
- Protects blood vessels.

Vitamin E d-alpha Tocopherol

- Prevents heart disease as anti-oxidant.

Earth Element of Chinese Medicine

Vitamin A

- Fortifies the lining of the Stomach.

Vitamin B-2 Riboflavin

- Associated with the Stomach's Yin qualities (cracks at the side of mouth, dry lips).
- Fortifies mucosa lining of Stomach-impacts sugar regulation & digestion.
- Impacts absorption of foods (symptom: undigested food in stool).

Vitamin B-6 Pantothenic Acid

- Supports the Spleen's function of metabolizing food.
- Supports the Spleen's function of extracting Qi energy from food (Symptom examples: Sinking Qi, muscle weakness).
- Deficiency associated with diabetes.

Vitamin B-6 Pyridoxine

- Associated with symptoms of Spleen Deficiency (feeling of heavy limbs, weak muscles, low energy-fatigue).
- Promotes the Spleen's function of assimilating foods (converts protein in to amino acids).

Vitamin B-7 Biotin

- Promotes the Spleen's function of assimilating foods (converts protein in to amino acids).
- Associated with symptoms of Spleen Deficiency (feeling of heavy limbs, weak muscles, low energy-fatigue).

Vitamin B-9 Folate

- Supports the Spleen function of generating tissue and promoting flesh.
- Protects Stomach Yin (mucosa lining).

Vitamin C Ascorbic Acid

- Enhances the Spleen's function of generating flesh-speeds healing from wounds and surgery.
- Resolves muscle fatigue.

Vitamin E d-alpha Tocopherol

Enhances the Spleen's function of generating flesh- speeds healing from wounds and surgery.

Metal Element of Chinese Medicine

The Metal Element of Chinese medicine includes the Lungs, Large Intestine, skin and sinuses. The Lungs are the most external Yin Organ in TCM and are closely associated with the Wei Qi which is associated with the immune response.

Vitamin A

- Benefits the skin.
- Enhances the ability to smell and taste.
- Protects the respiratory tract.
- Nourishes the mucous membranes of the Large Intestine & sinuses.
- Re-enforces the Wei Qi.

Vitamin B-1 Thiamine

- Benefits the Liver energetic organs ability to move Qi.

Vitamin B-3 Niacin

- Fortifies and thickens the skin.

Vitamin B-3 Niacin

- Combats dermatitis.

Vitamin C Ascorbic Acid

- Involved with bone growth.
- Treats all types of skin conditions.

Vitamin D-3 Cholecalciferol

- Protects the colon by enabling the lining to absorb calcium (possibly).

Vitamin E d-alpha Tocopherol

- Benefits the skin by maintaining the stability of skin membranes.
- Protects the Lungs from environmental toxins.

Brain (Sometimes referred to as a Curious Organ in Chinese Medicine)

- Vitamin B-1 Thiamine.
- Benefits neurological pathways (memory).
- Improves memory and concentration.
- Combats insomnia.

Vitamin B-3 Niacin

- Directs Qi and Blood up to the brain.

Vitamin B-3 Niacin

- Calms the Shen (necessary for psychological balances).

Vitamin B-6 Pyridoxine

- Used in children with autism (magnesium added to direct to the brain).

Vitamin B-7 Biotin

- Associated with unexplained mood disorders and mood swings.

Vitamin B-9 Folate

- Supports the utilization of amino acids in neurological structures of the brain.
- Supports bone marrow production (the Brain of Chinese medicine is the Sea of Marrow).

Vitamin B-12 Cobalamin

- Reinforces blood-brain barrier from toxins.
- Supports bone marrow production (the Brain of Chinese medicine is the Sea of Marrow).
- Deficiency results in a deterioration of neuro-connections.
- Associated with auto-immune disorders (think chron's disease).

Vitamin D-3 Cholecalciferol

- Improves mood (think seasonal disorder).

Vitamin E d-alpha Tocopherol

- Protects the membrane of the brain (think strokes).

The Three-Four Level Theory of Traditional Chinese Medicine

Theoretically, there are four levels that diseases must pass through; each becomes more serious as it progresses to deeper levels of the body. In reality, some viruses or diseases may not affect every level. This is a practical working theory of the most likely path that is taken:

- Wei (Defensive) Level.
- Qi Level (or stage).
- Ying (Nutritive) Level.
- Xue (Blood) Level.

Wei Qi Level

The Wei Qi level of Chinese medicine refers to the more outer-body protective abilities of the skin, nerves, muscles, sinews, tendons, and immune response (loosely). We have includes minerals and vitamins that play a role in the body's defenses beyond the immune system here also.

Vitamin A

- Tonifies the Wei Qi-bolsters the immune system.
- Protects the body from environmental toxins.

Vitamin B-1 Thiamine

- Benefits the nerves (neuropathy).
- Anti-oxidant.

Vitamin B-3 Niacin

- Fortifies and thickens the skin.

Vitamin B-6 Pyridoxine

- Affects neurological issues (carpal tunnel).

Vitamin B-7 Biotin

- Associated with neurological disorders (Parkinson's disease-peripheral neuropathy).

Vitamin B-9 Folate

- Used with cancer patients to rebuild healthy cellular division.

Vitamin B-12 Cobalamin

- Reinforces blood-brain barrier from toxins.
- Associated with auto-immune disorders when deficient.
- Deficiency results in a deterioration of nerve tissue (myelin sheath).

Vitamin C Ascorbic Acid

- Maintains the integrity of the skin.
- Defends against environmental toxins and stresses.
- Re-enforces immune system.
- Generates flesh and heals wounds.

Vitamin D-3 Cholecalciferol

- Boosts the immune system.

Vitamin E d-alpha Tocopherol

- Blocks the formation of tumors.
- Protects the lungs from environmental toxins.
- Protects the cells from environmental toxins and radiation.

Qi Level

At this stage, the disease has progressed into the interior and begins to reach the organs. We discussed individual organs in the Five Element theory archetype above.

Ying Qi Level

The Ying level of Chinese medicine is associated with the Blood, blood vessels, flesh, fascia, and connective tissue collectively.

Vitamin B-2 Riboflavin

- Promotes the production of red blood cells.
- Deficit of riboflavin associated with Blood Stagnation due to Blood Deficiency.

Vitamin B-3 Niacin

- Alleviates Blood Stagnation.
- Flushes, pushes out through the sensory organs of the head (skin, sinuses, eyes-think allergies).

Vitamin B-7 Biotin

- Resolves dermatological issues due to Heat in the Blood.

Vitamin B-9 Folate

- Promotes the production of health red blood cells.

Vitamin B-12 Cobalamin

- Protects blood vessels.

Vitamin C Ascorbic Acid

- Enhances the action of iron in the blood and Blood production.
- Anti-oxidant-cleanses the blood of damaging toxins.

Vitamin E d-alpha Tocopherol

- Reinforces the blood vessel walls.

Xue Level

This is the Blood Level where diseases and conditions become more serious. Heat in the Blood is a common manifestation.

Vitamin B-7 Biotin

- Used in conditions with Internal Wind (likely due to Liver Congestion-think Parkinson's disease).

Vitamin C Ascorbic Acid

- Lack of associated with bleeding gums.

Vitamin E d-alpha Tocopherol

- Powerful Blood level anti-oxidant (free radicals are Blood Heat).
- Prevents Blood Sticky (think cholesterol).

Yuan Qi Level

This is from yet another three-level system of Asian medicine that considers the Yuan level as the bone, marrow, genetic considerations (loosely the Kidney Jing or Essence), which would be the deepest level, or our core.

Vitamin B-9 Folate

- Promotes the DNA synthesis of cell division.
- Used with cancer patients preventatively with a familial history of cancer (think breast cancer).

Vitamin B-12 Cobalamin

- Plays a role in DNA synthesis.

Vitamin C Ascorbic Acid

- Involved with bone growth and collagen production.

Vitamin D-3 Cholecalciferol

- Facilitates the body's ability to utilize calcium in bone-building.

Vitamin E d-alpha Tocopherol

- Extends the life of cells and prevents aging.

List of Traditional Chinese Medicines

In Traditional Chinese Medicine, there are roughly 13,000 medicinals used in China and over 100,000 medicinal prescriptions recorded in the ancient literature. Plant elements and extracts are the most common elements used in medicines. In the classic Handbook of Traditional Drugs from 1941, 517 drugs were listed - 442 were plant parts, 45 were animal parts, and 30 were minerals.

Herbal medicine, as used in traditional Chinese medicine (TCM), came to widespread attention in the United States in the 1970s. At least 40 states in the United States license practitioners of Oriental medicine, and there are about 50 colleges of Oriental medicine in the United States today.

In Japan, the use of TCM herbs and herbal formulas is traditionally known as Kampo, literally "Han Chinese Medical Formulas". Many Kampo combinations are manufactured in Japan on a large scale by reputable manufacturers.

In Korea, more than 5000 herbs and 7000 herbal formulas are used in Traditional Korean Medicine for the prevention and treatment of ailments. These are herbs and formulas that are traditionally Korean or derived from, or are used in TCM.

In Vietnam, traditional medicine comprises Thuoc Bac (Northern Medicine) and Thuoc Nam (Southern Medicine). Only those who can understand Chinese characters could diagnose and prescribe remedies in Northern Medicine. The theory of Northern Medicine is based on the Yin-Yang interactions and the eight trigrams, as used in Chinese Medicine. Herbs such as Gleditsia sinensis are used in both Traditional Vietnamese Medicine and TCM.

Ginseng is the most broadly used substance for the most broad set of alleged cures. Powdered antlers, horns, teeth, and bones are second in importance to ginseng, with claims ranging from curing cancer to curing impotence.

Mammals

Human Parts and Excreta

Human body parts and excreta are currently used in TCM medicines and are included in its new textbooks and handbooks, such as licorice in human feces, dried human placenta, finger nails, child's urine, hair, and urinary sediments (Hominis Urinae Sedimentum, Ren Zhong Bai). The current consumption of human parts is considered cannibalism by some. Other parts include pubic hair, flesh, blood, bone, semen, and menstrual blood. The Bencao Gangmu describes the use of 35 human waste products and body parts as medicines, such as bones, fingernail, hairs, dandruff, earwax, impurities on the teeth, feces, urine, sweat, and organs. - Also listed are human breath and the "soul of criminals that were hanged", which is considered under TCM to be a material object resembling charcoal that is dug out of the ground beneath the body shortly after a hanged criminal died, but very few human or allegedly human products remain in use today.

There is considerable controversy about the ethics of use of criminals for body parts, using humans as commodities, and consumption of human body parts which some consider to be cannibalism.

Dried Human Placenta

Dried human placenta is believed to treat male impotence, male and female infertility, chronic cough, asthma, and insomnia.

Human Feces and Urine

The contemporary use of licorice in prepared human feces is known as Ren Zhong Huang Human urine sediment is called Ren Zhong Bai. Both Ren Zhong Huang and Ren Zhong Bai are used to treat inflammatory conditions and fungal infections of the skin and mouth.

In Traditional Chinese medicine, human feces is used in a decoction of licorice. These feces-licorice decoctions have been found to have profound differences in pharmacokinetics as compared to pure glycyrrhizin. Initial studies investigating traditional Chinese

Medicine indicate that taking the fecal bacteria alongside the licorice may improve the pharmacokinetics of glycyrrhizin, and certain strains of gut bacteria may produce an anti-tumor effect and an immune boosting effect. Human gut flora may protect against cell damage caused by hydrogen peroxide.

Human Penis

> "The human penis is not a drug."
>
> — Li Shizhen

Human penis is believed under TCM to stop bleeding, and as with other TCM medicines, the basis for belief in its therapeutic effects is anecdotal and not based on the scientific method; Li Shizhen, author of the greatest pharmacological work in pre-modern China, the Bencao Gangmu, objected to use of human penis, but cited the anecdotal evidence and included it in the Bencao Gangmu, which is still a standard reference today.

Human Pubic Hair

Human pubic hair ("shady hair") was claimed to cure snakebite, difficult birth, abnormal urination, and "yin and yang disorder" (A disease unique to TCM based on its views of sexual behavior).

Donkey-Hide Gelatin

Gelatin made from the hide of donkeys (ejiao) is made into pellets for use in making teas.

Deer Penis

Deer penis is commonly sold in Chinese pharmacies. and served in specialized restaurants such as the Guo Li Zhuang restaurant in Beijing. The deer penis is typically very large and, under TCM it must be extracted from the deer whilst still alive. Often it is then sliced into small pieces, typically by women and then roasted and dried in the sun and then preserved while the deer looks on.China banned deer penis wine during the 2008 Summer Olympics, as it is believed that the wine is an effective treatment for athletic injuries.

Flying Squirrel Feces

Flying Squirrel Feces is used to Stop Bleeding.

The text Chinese Medical Herbology and Pharmacology notes that flying squirrel feces has a "distinct odor" that "may decrease patient compliance" with ingesting it.

It is believed to have uses for amenorrhea, menses pain, postpartum abdominal pain, epigastric pain, and chest pain. It is boiled in a decoction with other herbs prior to ingestion. If it is to be used in a formula to stop heavy bleeding; it is dry fried prior to making the decoction. Exposure to flying squirrel feces in the wild has been associated with Rickettsia infections.

Pangolin Scales

Scales of pangolins are used in traditional Chinese medicine.

Rhinoceros Horn

The horn of a rhinoceros is used as an antipyretic - because it is believed to "cool the blood" - however several scientific studies failed to find any active antipyretic molecule in rhinoceros horn. The illegal trade in rhinoceros horns has decimated the world's rhino population by more than 90 percent over the past 40 years.

Tiger Penis

The penis and testicles of male tigers is used by some to treat erectile dysfunction and to improve sexual performance, despite tiger penis being a placebo. Critically endangered species such as the Sumatran tiger are often being hunted to keep up with the illegal demand for tiger parts.

Reptiles and Amphibians

Snake Oil

Snake oil is the most widely known Chinese medicine in the west, due to extensive marketing in the west in the late 1800s and early 1900s, and wild claims of its efficacy to treat many maladies. Snake oil is a traditional Chinese medicine used to treat joint pain by rubbing it on joints as a liniment.

This is theoretically possible because snake oil is higher in eicosapentaenoic acid than most other oils. But there are no scientific studies showing that rubbing it on joints has any positive effect, or that snake oil is safe for daily consumption.

Toad Secretions

The secretions of various species of toads are an ingredient in certain traditional Chinese teas. However, these teas may contain deadly amounts of cardiac glycosides and thus should be avoided.

Toad-headed Gecko

Toad-head geckos are gutted, beheaded, dried and then crushed, and are used to treat asthma, male impotence and the common cold.

Turtle Shell

Widespread medicinal use of turtle shells is of concern to conservationists.

Marine Life

- Seahorse: Seahorse (Hai Ma) is a fundamental ingredient in therapies for a variety of disorders, including asthma, arteriosclerosis, incontinence, impotence, insomnia, thyroid disorders, skin ailments, broken bones, heart disease, throat infections, abdominal pain, sores, skin infections; it is also used as an aphrodisiac and to facilitate childbirth. As many as 20 million seahorses per year may be used for TCM purposes. In one study, 58 seahorse samples were collected from various TCM vendors in Taiwan, and of all the eight species identified from the fifty-eight samples, seven were vulnerable, and one was endangered.
- Shark Fin Soup: Shark fin soup is traditionally regarded as beneficial for health in East Asia, and its status as an elite dish has led to huge demand with the increase of affluence in China, devastating shark populations.

Insects

- Blister Beetle: Blister beetles (Ban mao) are believed under TCM to treat skin lesions, because they cause them. They contain the blister agent cantharidin.
- Centipede: Powdered centipede (wu gong) is believed under TCM to treat tetanus, seizures, convulsions, skin lesions, and pain. It is toxic.
- Hornets Nest: Hornets nest (lu feng fang) is used to treat skin disorders and ringworm. It may be toxic.
- Leech: Hirudo medicinalis is used in TCM to treat amenorrhea, abdominal and chest pain, and constipation.
- Scorpion: Dried scorpions may be ground into a powder and mixed with water. In TCM, powdered scorpion is toxic and is therefore used to treat poisoning. A scorpion venom peptide was found to help with arthritis in vitro.
- Fungi: Various fungi are used in TCM. Some may have scientifically proven medicinal value, while others may be extremely toxic.

Supernatural Mushroom

The supernatural mushroom (lingzhi mushroom, Chinese "linh chi" = "supernatural mushroom", "reishi mushroom" in Japan) encompasses several fungal species of the genus Ganoderma, and most commonly refers to the closely related species, Ganoderma lucidum and Ganoderma tsugae. G. lucidum enjoys special veneration in East Asia, where it has been used as a medicinal mushroom in traditional Chinese medicine for more than 2,000 years, making it one of the oldest mushrooms known to have been used medicinally. Today, the ling zhi mushroom is used in a herbal formula designed to minimize the side effects of chemotherapy.

Extracts of the mushroom are used as a commercial pharmaceutical to suppress cancer cell proliferation and migration, although the mechanisms by which this is achieved are currently unknown.

Tremella Fuciformis

Tremella fuciformis is used as a beauty product by women in China and Japan as it reportedly increases moisture retention in the skin and prevents senile degradation of micro-blood vessels in the skin, reducing wrinkles and smoothing fine lines. Other beneficial effects come from its ability to increase the activity of SOD in the brain and liver.

Plants

There are thousands of plants that are used as medicines. The following list represents a very small portion of the TCM pharmacopoeia.

Aconite

Monkshood root is commonly used in TCM. It was once so commonly used it was called "the king of the 100 herbs".

The monkshood plant contains what is called "the queen of poisons", the highly toxic alkaloid aconitine. Aconitine is easily absorbed through the skin, eyes and through the lining of the nose; Death may occur through respiratory paralysis. A few minutes after exposure, paresthesia starts at the mouth and slowly beings to cover the whole body, Anesthesia, hot and cold flashes, nausea and vomiting and other similar symptoms follow. Sometimes there is strong pain, accompanied by cramps, or diarrhea.

When a person has a negative reaction to the alkaloid, some practitioners of classical Chinese medicine think that this is because it was that the monkshood plant was processed incorrectly or planted on the wrong place or on the wrong day of the year; Not because of an overdose

The Chinese also used aconitine both for hunting and for warfare.

Birthworts

Birthworts (family Aristolochiaceae) are often used to treat many aliments, including hypertension, hemorrhoids, and colic. However - they are of little medicinal value and contain the carcinogen aristolochic acid. The over-use of this plant family in TCM is thought be a significant cause of upper urinary tract cancer and kidney failure in Taiwan; in 2012, approximately a third of all herbal prescriptions in Taiwan contained AA. Supplements containing AA may be responsible for BEN.

Camellia Sinensis

Tea from India, Sri Lanka, Java and Japan is used in TCM for aches and pains, digestion, depression, detoxification, as an energizer and, to prolong life.

Cayenne Pepper

Cayenne pepper is believed under TCM to be a prophylactic medicine.

Chinese Cucumber

The fruit of Trichosanthes kirilowii is believed to treat tumors, reduce fevers, swelling and coughing, abscesses, amenorrhea, jaundice, and polyuria. The plant is deadly if improperly prepared; causing pulmonary edema, cerebral hemorrhage, seizures, and high fever.

Chrysanthemum Flowers

Chrysanthemum flowers (Ju Hua) are used in TCM to treat headaches, fever, dizziness and dry eyes. They are also used to make certain beverages. Chrysanthemum flowers are believed to "brighten the eyes, pacify the liver, break blood, clear heat, stop dysentery, disperse wind, relieve toxicity, and regulate the center".

Cocklebur Fruit

Cocklebur fruit (Xanthium, cang er zi) is one of the most important herbs in TCM, and is commonly to treat sinus congestion, chronic nasal obstructions and discharges, and respiratory allergies.

The plant is mildly toxic and can cause gastrointestinal upset.

Crow Dipper

Pinellia ternata is believed under TCM to be the strongest of all TCM herbs for removing phlegm.

Active ingredinets of this herb include: methionine, glycine, β-aminobutyric acid, γ-aminobutyric acid, ephedrine, trigonelline, phytosterols and glucoronic acid.

Care should be taken as crow dipper is toxic.

Croton Seed

Seeds of Croton tiglium are used in TCM to treat gastrointestinal disorders, convulsions, and skin lesions. They are often used with rhubarb, dried ginger and apricot seed. Care should be taken as the seeds are toxic and carcinogenic.

Dioscorea Root

In TCM, Dioscorea Root (Radix Dioscorea, Huai Shan Yao or Shan Yao in Chinese), benefits both the Yin and Yang, and is used to tonify the lungs, spleen and kidney. It can "be used in large amounts and 30g is suggested when treating diabetes". If taken habitually, it "brightens the intellect and prolongs life".

Ginger

Ginger root, Zingiber officinale, has been used in China for over 2,000 years to treat indigestion, upset stomach, diarrhea, and nausea. It is also used in TCM to treat arthritis, colic, diarrhea, heart conditions, the common cold, flu-like symptoms, headaches, and menstrual cramps. Today, health care professionals worldwide commonly recommend ginger to help prevent or treat nausea and vomiting associated with motion sickness, pregnancy, and cancer chemotherapy. It is also used as a treatment for minor stomach upset, as a supplement for arthritis, and may even help prevent heart disease and cancer.

Ginkgo

Ginkgo biloba seeds are crushed and believed under TCM to treat asthma. G. biloba has been used by humans for nearly 5,000 years. However, further scientific studies are needed to establish the efficacy of G. biloba as a medicine.

Ginseng

Ginseng root is the most widely sold traditional Chinese medicine. The name "ginseng" is used to refer to both American (Panax quinquefolius) and Asian or Korean ginseng (P. ginseng), which belong to the species Panax and have a similar chemical makeup. Siberian ginseng or Eleuthero (Eleutherococcus senticosus) is another type of plant. Asian ginseng has a light tan, gnarled root that often looks like a human body with stringy shoots for arms and legs. In ancient times, herbalists thought that because of the way ginseng looks it could treat many different kinds of syndromes, from fatigue and stress to asthma and cancer. In traditional Chinese medicine, ginseng was often combined with other herbs and used often to bring longevity, strength, and mental alacrity to its users. Asian ginseng is believed to enhance the immune system in preventing and treating infection and disease. Several clinical studies report that

Asian ginseng can improve immune function. Studies have found that ginseng seems to increase the number of immune cells in the blood, and improve the immune system's response to a flu vaccine. In one study, 227 participants received either ginseng or placebo for 12 weeks, with a flu shot administered after 4 weeks. The number of colds and flu were two-thirds lower in the group that took ginseng.

Ginseng contains stimulants, but may produce side effect including high blood pressure, low blood pressure, and mastalgia. Ginseng may also lead to induction of mania in depressed patients who mix it with antidepressants. One of the most common and characteristic symptoms of acute overdose of ginseng from the genus Panax is bleeding. Symptoms of mild overdose with Panax ginseng may include dry mouth and lips, excitation, fidgeting, irritability, tremor, palpitations, blurred vision, headache, insomnia, increased body temperature, increased blood pressure, edema, decreased appetite, increased sexual desire, dizziness, itching, eczema, early morning diarrhea, bleeding, and fatigue. Symptoms of gross overdose with Panax ginseng may include nausea, vomiting, irritability, restlessness, urinary and bowel incontinence, fever, increased blood pressure, increased respiration, decreased sensitivity and reaction to light, decreased heart rate, cyanotic facial complexion, red face, seizures, convulsions, and delirium.

The constituents of ginseng include triterpene saponins, aglycone protopanaxadiol, aglycone protopanaxytriol, aglycone oleanolic acid and water-soluble polysaccharides.

Goji Berry

Marketing literature for goji berry (wolfberry) products including several "goji juices" suggest that wolfberry polysaccharides have extensive biological effects and health benefits, although none of these claims have been supported by peer-reviewed research.

A May 2008 clinical study published by the peer-reviewed Journal of Alternative and Complementary Medicine indicated that parametric data, including body weight, did not show significant differences between subjects receiving Lycium barbarum berry juice and subjects receiving the placebo; the study concluded that subjective measures of health were improved and suggested further research in humans was necessary. This study, however, was subject to a variety of criticisms concerning its experimental design and interpretations.

Published studies have also reported possible medicinal benefits of Lycium barbarum, especially due to its antioxidant properties, including potential benefits against cardiovascular and inflammatory diseases, vision-related diseases (such as age-related macular degeneration and glaucoma), having neuroprotective properties or as an anticancer and immunomodulatory agent.

Wolfberry leaves may be used to make tea, together with Lycium root bark (called dìg ǔ pí in Chinese), for traditional Chinese medicine (TCM). A glucopyranoside isolated from wolfberry root bark have inhibitory activity in vitro against human pathogenic bacteria and fungi.

Horny Goat Weed

Horny goat weed (Yin Yang Huo,) may have use in treating erectile dysfunction. Exploitation of wild populations may have a serious impact on the surrounding environment.

Lily Bulb

Lily bulbs (Bai He) are used in TCM to treat dry cough, dry and sore throat, and wheezing.

Chinese Rhubarb

The root of "Chinese rhubarb," or "da huang," either Rheum palmatum, or Rheum officinale, is an important herb that is used primarily as a laxative in Chinese Traditional Medicine. The degree of potency depends on how long the root is cooked during preparation after harvesting.

Round Cardamon Fruit

Round cardamon fruit (Bai Dou Kou) is used in TCM to treat poor appetite, breathing problems, vomiting and diarreahea.

Thunder God Vine

Thunder god vine is used in TCM to treat arthritis, relieve pain and reduce joint swelling. It can be extremely toxic, if not processed properly If used inappropriately, within two to three hours after ingestion, a patient may begin to have diarrhea, headache, dizziness, severe vomiting (sometimes with blood), chills, high fever, and irregular heart beat. Long term inproper use may result in nervous system damage.

Trichosanthis Root

In TCM, Trichosanthis Root (Radix Trichosanthis or Tian Hua Fen in Chinese), is used to clear heat, generate fluids when heat injures fluids causing thirst, in the wasting and thirsting syndrome. The pairing of Tian Hua Fen and Zhi Mu had a faster, stronger and longer effect in reducing blood sugar levels than either herb alone.

Strychnine Tree Seed

The seeds of the Strychnine tree, Strychnos nux-vomica, are sometimes used to treat diseases of the respiratory tract, anemia, and geriatric complaints. The active molecule is strychnine, a compound often used as a pesticide. Strychnine can also be used as a stimulant - however it has an extremely low therapeutic index and better, less toxic replacements are available.

Sweet Wormwood

Sweet wormwood (Artemisia annua, Qing Hao) is believed under TCM to treat fever, headache, dizziness, stopping bleeding, and alternating fever and chills.

Sweet wormwood had fallen out of common use under TCM until it was rediscovered in the 1970s when the Chinese Handbook of Prescriptions for Emergency Treatments was found. This pharmacopeia contained recipes for a tea from dried leaves, prescribed for fevers (not specifically malaria). The plant extracts often used in TCM are antimalarial, due to the presence of artemisinin.

However, it has been questioned as to whether tea made from A. annua is effective against malaria, since artemesinin is not soluble in water and the resulting tea would not be expected to contain any significant amount of artemesinin.

Willow Bark

Plants of the genus Salix have been used since the time of Hippocrates when patients were advised to chew on the bark to reduce fever and inflammation. Willow bark has been used throughout the centuries in China and Europe to the present for the treatment of pain (particularly low back pain and osteoarthritis), headache, and inflammatory conditions such as bursitis and tendinitis. The bark of white willow contains salicin, which is a chemical similar to aspirin (acetylsalicylic acid). It is thought to be responsible for the pain-relieving and anti-inflammatory effects of the herb. In 1829, salicin was used to develop aspirin. White willow appears to be slower than aspirin to bring pain relief, but its effects may last longer.

Minerals

Arsenic

Arsenic sulfide (Xiong Huang) is a toxic mineral used in TCM to kill parasitic worms and treat sore throats, swellings, abscesses, itching, rashes, and malaria.

Arsenic, while possibly essential for life in tiny amounts, is extremely toxic in the amounts used and arsenic poisoning may result from improper use of arsenic containing remedies. They are most commonly given as a pill or capsule, although are sometimes incorporated into a mixture with other substances.

Lead

Galena is used in TCM to treat ringworm, skin disorders and ulcers, and is thought to "detoxify" the body. It is crushed and taken orally or used on the skin. Lead tetroxide (Qian Dan) is used to treat anxiety, itching, and malaria. It is important to note that most lead compounds are extremely toxic.

Mercury

Cinnabar

Despite its toxicity, mercury sulfide (cinnabar) has historically been used in Chinese medicine, where it is called zhūshā and was highly valued in Chinese Alchemy. It was also referred to as dān meaning all of Chinese alchemy, cinnabar, and the "elixir of immortality". Cinnabar has been used in Traditional Chinese medicine as a sedative for more than 2000 years, and has been shown to have sedative and toxic effects in mice. In addition to being used for insomnia, cinnabar is thought to be effective for cold sores, sore throat, and some skin infections.

Corrosive Sublimate

Mercury (II) chloride (Qing Fen) is used in TCM to "detoxify" the body, kill intestinal parasites, and as a mild tranquilizer.

HUMAN BIOLOGICAL RHYTHM IN TRADITIONAL CHINESE MEDICINE

The thought of "harmony between human and nature" is rooted in traditional Chinese philosophy and a conclusion about the relationship between people and the nature, highly generalized by ancient Chinese. In TCM, this thought is the logical basis for understanding human biology and pathology and contains three connotations. Firstly it is the isomorphism between human and nature, i.e., their compatibility on structure and composition. It was stated in Keqi of Spiritual Pivot that five Zang organs of human compatible with five musical scales of heaven, six Fu organs of human compatible with six tunes of heaven, 365 acupoints of human compatible with 365 days a year; knees and shoulders of human compatible with mountains on the land; axilla and popliteal spaces of human compatible with valleys on land; 12 meridians of man compatible with 12 rivers on the land, etc. Similarly, the rhythm of nature can be also observed in human body. Therefore, isomorphism between human and nature is a TCM explanation of the presence of biological rhythms. Secondly there are same virtues between human and nature, i.e., there are similar and comparable functions and phenomenon between human and nature. It was stated in Tianyuanji Article of Plain Questions that human has five Zang organs that can metabolize five Qi to generate happiness, anger, thoughts, sorrow and dread, just like the heaven has Five Elements that can drive Five Positions to generate coldness, heat, dryness, wetness and wind. Visceral manifestation theory in TCM is centered on the understanding of functions of heart, liver, spleen, lung and kidney of human body via natural phenomenon of generation, growth, metabolism, collection and storage, relating temporal factors like day, night and four seasons to biological and pathological variations.

Same virtues between human and the heaven, therefore, are the main theoretical basis and main approaches in investigation on biological rhythms in TCM.

Thirdly it is interaction between human and heaven, i.e., as the individual system of its own, human and nature are open but not closed, with mutual exchange of information and energy and mutual influences. It was stated in Yinyangyingxiang Article of Plain Questions that Heaven Qi is communicated to Lung, Earth Qi to throat, Wind Qi to Liver, Thunder Qi to Heart, Grain Qi to Spleen and Rain Qi to Kidney. It is also a prerequisite of explaining human pathological rhythms in TCM, as stated in Zangqifashi Article of Plain Questions that a patient with liver diseases feels fresh in the morning, but the disease tends to be aggravated in the evening and then relieved at midnight. It is also a basic foundation for TCM health care, as stated in Siqitiaoshen Article of Plain Questions that the sage cultivates his Yang during spring and summer and his Yin during autumn and winter. Interaction between human and heaven is the theoretical foundation and approaches to apply biological rhythm to practice.

In summary, based on the point of views in TCM, biological rhythms are inherent biological functions analogous to natural rhythms, and can be intervened through some positive approaches.

Biological Rhythms in TCM Theory

Given the fact of harmony between human and the heaven, all rhythms in the nature should be found in human body! In fact, in comparison with modern medicine scrutinizing circadian rhythms but neglecting other rhythms, Huangdi's Canon of Medicine description about circadian rhythm, syzygial rhythm and seasonal rhythm is of great reference value in details.

Human circadian rhythm is embodied in the operation of Ying Qi and Wei Qi, as stated in Yingweishenghui Article of Spiritual Pivot that Ying Qi circulates within pulse and Wei Qi circulates out of pulse, and they circulate continuously, Ying Qi has the circulating rule of fifty cycles along the body within one day and one night, Wei Qi has the rule of circulating along yang (the external body) during daytime for 25 circles and yin (the internal body) during night for 25 circles, the circulation of Wei-qi dominates human sleeping/awake cycle. Moreover, it is put forward by Shunqiyirifenweisishi Article of Spiritual Pivot the rhythm division method imitating four seasons that one day is divided into four seasons with morning as the spring, noon as the summer, sunset as the fall and midnight as the winter. Similarly, human also has the biological rhythm that qi emerges in the morning, grows at the noon, declines in the evening and enters organs at midnight, which is analogous to seasonal rhythms with its significance listed as following.

Human syzygial rhythm is embodied in prosperity-decline variation of qi and blood. It is stated in Bazhengshenming Article of Plain Questions that accumulation of blood qi and circulation of Wei Qi start from crescent; at the full moon, blood qi are substantiated and muscles strengthened; at the wane, muscles and meridians are weakened,

Wei Qi is gone and figure exists alone without essence. It is stated in Suilu Article of Spiritual Pivot that at the full moon sea water flushes to the west and human qi and blood are accumulated with strengthened muscles, tight skin, strong hair and compact texture, but at the wane sea water flushes to the east and human qi and blood are weak, with Wei Qi gone, figure alone (without essence), shrunk muscles, flabby skin, open texture, sparse hair and thin muscle texture. So phase of the moon is synchronized with the prosperity-decline of human blood and qi.

Human seasonal rhythms are the biological rhythm that is discussed most in Huangdi's Canon of Medicine, and is embodied in rotated duties of Five Zang organs. Liver is on duty in spring, heart in summer, lung in autumn and kidney in winter. Due to Five Zang organs taking turns to be on duty, pulse manifestation also shows periodical changes including pulse in spring like string, summer flood, autumn hair and winter stone; based on which human also show corresponding vulnerability to certain diseases. The rhythm that Five Zang organs take turn on duty is the most important idea concerning rhythm in TCM. It should be pointed out that human seasonal rhythm contains a group of complex causalities, is fulfilled through highly orderly cooperation between multiple function of creatures, and is hard to understand if a single causality is isolated. That's probably why few modern biological researches aim at the seasonal rhythm.

Concerning human seasonal rhythm, there are many other patterns of rhythms in Huangdi's Canon of Medicine besides the rule of Five Zang taking turns to be on duty. For example, it is stated in Zhenyaojingzhong Article of Plain Questions that human qi is in liver at lunar month 1 and 2, in spleen at lunar month 3 and 4, at head at lunar month 5 and 6, at lung at lunar month 7 and 8, at heart at lunar month 9 and 10, and at kidney at lunar month 11 and 12. It is stated in Yinyangxiriyue Article of Spiritual Pivot a rhythm model that twelve meridians in feet correspond to the 12 months. Moreover, besides the significant biological rhythms of day, month and year, 10-day rhythm is also recorded in Huangdi's Canon of Medicine. Despite fewer articles are for this rhythm, it can be applied to prognosis and evaluation of diseases.

Among all these three rhythms, circadian rhythm and seasonal rhythm are especially focused on by TCM, and discussion and application of Syzygial rhythm seem fewer.

Yin-Yang and Five Elements are the Theories and Methods for Investigation on Biological Rhythm in TCM

Yin-yang and Five Elements Theory, based on Theory of qi monism, is the most important theoretical utensil for TCM. Yin Yang and Five Elements Theory is still applied generally to understanding of the phenomena of biological rhythm.

Yin-yang is used in Huangdi's Canon of Medicine to understand circadian rhythm. It is stated in Jinhuizhenyan Article of Plain Questions that one day consists of day (yang) and night (yin), and the day and night could also divided into two periods, yang and yin. The period from early morning to noon is "yang (the first half) of yang (day)", from noon to evening is "yin of yang", from evening to crow is "yin of yin" and from crow to early morning is "yang of yin". Four periods during one day and one night have their yin and yang features respectively. Instantly after yin and yang of a nature day is discussed, it is followed by a statement of "therefore human should comply with it". How should human being comply with the nature? It lies in yin yang profile endowed to Five Zang organs including heart as the Yang of Yang, lung as the Yin of Yang, kidney as Yin of Yin, liver as Yang of Yin, and spleen as the utmost Yin of Yin.

A certain correlation can be established between a period and an organ with the same features. Due to the similarity in locations and functions in subject of their own, human circadian rhythm can be divided into four stages including "yang of yin, to yang of yang, to yin of yang, and to yin of yin" also named as "Shaoyang, Taiyang, Taiyin and Shaoyin". We can utilize yin yang features to carry out research and applications.

Take the heart as the example, heart takes its turn on duty from early morning to noon. Research reveal that blood pressure and heart rate reach to the peaks during this period in a day, and so does the incidence of heart diseases such as myocardial infarction, arrhythmia, angina pectoris and sudden cardiac death.1 From the point of view in TCM, the whole body is in a state of "yang of yang" during the natural state of "yang of yang". Heart is the executor of this state, so the requirement on heart by body seems most urgent, cardiac burden rises to the highest point, and risks of exhausted heart qi seems the highest with the highest incidence of morbidity.

Taking turn on duty by "liver–heart–lung–kidney" is the essence of quartation of day–night rhythm, it can be inferred that lung diseases most likely occur on the afternoon with risk of aggravation and death; kidney diseases from evening to midnight, and liver diseases from midnight to sun rise. It has been confirmed that severe liver disease (including severe viral hepatitis, decompensated liver cirrhosis and hepatocellular carcinoma) has the highest mortality during the latter half of the night, and the period from 15 to 19 o'clock (Shenyou Period) witnesses the highest death rate of lung cancer patient, which seems consistent with conclusion in TCM, reflecting the accuracy of understanding of biological circadian rhythm in TCM.

TCM uses mainly Five Element Theory to understand seasonal rhythm, and each season has its "Five-Element feature" of its own, such as spring corresponding to wood, summer to fire, long summer to soil, autumn to gold, and winter to water. Similarly, Five Zang organs also have their "Five-Element features" respectively, such as liver belonging to wood, heart to fire, spleen to earth, lung to metal and kidney to water. Therefore, human body appears a seasonal rhythm of rotating duty by "liver–heart–spleen–lung–kidney" similar to the natural rhythm, as stated in Zangqifashi Article of Plain Questions that liver dominates spring, heart summer, spleen long summer, lung autumn and kidney winter. Therefore, we can use Five Element Theory to investigate and apply human seasonal rhythm.

How can human seasonal rhythm be expressed? The accurate expression is variation in pulse manifestation. In Yujizhenyao Article of Plain Questions, a periodic variation of "spring pulse like string", "summer pulse like hook", "autumn pulse like floats" and "winter pulse like stone", which reflect the state of qi and blood, and therefore human blood and qi during four seasons also appear periodic variation.

Unfortunately, qi blood is hard to visualize, and activity of qi is difficult to normalize and standardize, so the biological seasonal rhythms are hard to represent with symbolic events. However, it does not mean that it is unknowable. Indeed the seasonal rhythms of onset of diseases can reflect from the side view the biological season rhythms. For example, spring is the season of high incidence of depression. This can be elucidated based on syndrome differentiation of Zang-Fu organs, in that the syndrome differentiated in TCM is positioned at liver with a deficiency feature in the depression patient, spring belongs to wood and orders of genesis and growth dominate, then the whole body needs to enter "wood" state relying on the genesis and growth function of liver. Therefore, in the case of liver deficiency, body requirement can not be satisfied and exterior requirement may in turn aggravate exhaustion of liver qi, resulting in depression state with the failure of body's entry into "genesis and growth" rhythm.

Additional research have confirmed that incidence of liver cancer in spring is higher than that in other seasons. It can be inferred that rhythm of disease onset can be adopted as the indirect proof for presence of human biological rhythms. It should be noted that human rhythm of "liver–heart–spleen–lung–kidney" is absolutely not a sequential prosperity-decline cycle of a single organ in turn, but a rhythm with successive appearance of states of "wood–fire–soil–gold–water" in whole body, "a certain organ is on duty" is only a description because a specific organ is needed during a specific period to exert the function to accomplish the changes of rhythm.

In summary, the connotation of rhythm either circadian or seasonal is a continuous variation in functional state of human body during a day or a year. During a specific period human body may be in a specific state, and there should be transition and continuity between different stages. Theories of Yin Yang and Five Elements are both the language tools to describe the state and theoretical tools applied to investigation of the states. Five Zang organs play an important role in the conversion and realization of functional stages. If this connotation is understood, it is easy to comprehend the difference between dichotomy, quartation and five-equal partition, and it is the most reasonable method as long as it describes accurately the feature in that stage, just like multiple expressions are used for a same stage in Huangdi's Canon of Medicine, sometimes with Yin Yang and sometimes with Five Elements.

Destruction of Biological Rhythm is in the Scope of Etiology in TCM

Biological rhythm is one of human biological functions, and failure of fulfillment of this function may cause disease. It is stated in Tiaojing Article of Plain Questions that the genesis of evil is from yin (internal factors) or yang (external factors), that from yang is caused by wind, rain, cold and heat, while that from yin is caused by food, domicile, and extreme emotion like happiness and anger. It points out that food intake without abstention and regular time and non-regular daily lives are some reasons for genesis of disease evils, with the mechanism that abnormal intake and living habits destroy normal rhythms of human being, thereby causing imbalance between yin and yang, bias in Five Elements, and finally, the morbidity.

It is proved by research that destruction of biological rhythm may induce or accelerate onset of multiple diseases, broken wake-sleeping rhythm is an important factor inducing Alzheimer's disease, disturbance of circadian rhythm caused by light pollution during night or shift work may induce disorder in metabolism and therefore cause multiple diseases such as obesity, diabetes and metabolic syndromes, and is a risk factor for breast cancer. Moreover, the stability in human biological rhythm may decrease along with the increase in age. Still other research have confirmed that destroyed human rhythm is a factor that can not be ignored during the pathogenesis of cardiovascular diseases and chronic diseases such as cancers. Therefore, more and more attention is being paid to working patterns or systems contradicted to human rhythms in modern society, as one of pathogens. A new round of revolution is being triggered in some of the fields to conform to human biological rhythms.

Modern medicine prioritizes the physical changes happening firstly and then inducing functional abnormality, and attributes the latter to the former, resulting in an explanation of diseases in a more and more microscopic point of view. On the contrary, TCM emphasizes the invisible destruction of functions inducing physical lesion and attributes physical alteration to disorder in human qi activity. Therefore, TCM adopts a comprehensive point-of-view of "time–space–human" to elucidate diseases, and thereby having much more advantages in understanding biological rhythms in a whole point of view.

Maintenance of Biological Rhythms is the Important Part in TCM Health Care

Biological rhythm is the biological function of human body, and it is considered in TCM that physical fitness with longevity can be realized as long as this function is maintained at the normal level. Shanggutianzhen Article of Plain Questions argues that ancients who knew the truth imitating yin yang and being consistent with the fluctuation of yin and yang, with good habit in food intake and living, without over working, so he could live his full span of one hundred years after termination of both figure and essence, and would not die until 100 years old. This article emphasizes especially the significance of good habit in food intake and living. It is recorded in Shengqitongtian Article of Plain Questions that stopping work in the twilight without disturbance of bones and muscles, avoid external evils as fog or dew, which can be adopted as commandment in maintenance of circadian rhythm. Siqitiaoshen Article of Plain Questions argues the guideline on living during four seasons, with spring as the example, one should sleep and gets up early, walk around within the park with hair disheveled to generate ambition. This also contains guidelines managing one's emotion.

The statement of "The alternation of day and night, and the circle of four seasons, are the laws that everything must obey, and the fundamental of life activity, the revolt against it should result in disasters, and obedience to it prevent from diseases" expresses emphasis on biological rhythm in TCM and its application, which is one of vital theories in TCM. Under the style of "future medicine", new glories will be shined by the health care principle in TCM centered on maintaining biological rhythms.

Application of Biological Rhythm to Treatments in TCM

In TCM treatment, the theory of biological rhythms is put into effect thoroughly. The usage of acupuncture emphasizes the "simulation of time", the acupoint-selection principle is different in different seasons, Xing acupoints are taken in spring, Shu acupoints in summer, He acupoints in autumn and Jing acupoints and Shu acupoints in winter. That is the acupoint-selection principle based on seasonal rhythms.

It is stated in Bazhengshenming Article of Plain Questions that no reducing therapy should be used at the crescent, no supplement at the full moon, and no treatment at the wane, which is an acupuncture principle based on Syzygial rhythm. The application of human biological rhythm is also embodied in method of acupoint selection according to theory of midnight-noon and ebb-flow.

Attention is also paid to obedience to human rhythm when using TCM prescription. For example, it is stated in Distinguish between Vomiting of Treatise on Cold-Induced Disease that the truth is that emetic therapy is suitable for spring, that is to say, it yields twice the result with half the effort if emetic therapy is used to treat disease in obedience to the qi activities in spring. In modern medicine, biological rhythm has also been considered when a regimen is being established,11 for example, treatment for high blood pressure based on the principle to re-establish circadian rhythm of blood pressure, and usage of chemotherapy for tumors based on rhythm of tumor growth. TCM is the pioneer in this regard.

Difficulties in Understandings of Biological Rhythms in TCM

Still, some difficulties exist in understandings of biological rhythms in TCM. Firstly, there is no a unified pattern correlating time division to organs. In day–night division pattern of Tai Shao Yin Yang, spleen is not referred to but only liver, heart, lung and kidney, and there are two different patterns in seasonal division: that of four seasons and that of five seasons, corresponding to two different opinions in Five Organs Theory of that "spleen dominates last 18 days of four seasons" (spleen does not dominate a certain season) and of "spleen dominates the long summer". Therefore, the effect of spleen in biological rhythm seems relatively vague.

Secondly, there are different concepts of disease rhythms in Huangdi's Canon of Medicine, and the applicable scope of various concepts and their accuracy seem inexact. There is an Article about "healing, aggravation, elimination and persistence" on five organ diseases in Zangqifashi Article of Plain Questions, take kidney as the example, "for the disease of kidney, healing is in spring; if not healed in spring, it aggravates in long summer; it is not eliminated in long summer, persists in hidden state during autumn, and ameliorates in winter"; "for kidney disease, it is relieved at midnight, aggravates during the hours of Chen, Xu, Chou and Wei (12 h timing method in ancient China), but persists on afternoon. For example, research have suggested that spring, summer and autumn are the seasons with high incidence of IgA nephropathy in Sichuan Province, with peak of average rate of admission is on June 12th while winter is the season with low incidence, which is consistent with the description in TCM that kidney disease is severe during long summer and ameliorates in winter. However, the epidemiology of mortality in lung cancer reported by Wei Wang et al. seems not consistent with the statement in the Zangqifashi Article of Plain Questions that lung disease is eliminated in summer, ameliorates in autumn, ameliorates on afternoon and aggravates at noon, but consistent with corresponding theories stated in Truth Theory of Golden Chamber. Therefore, the different theories found in Huangdi's Canon of Medicine need further elucidation and clarification.

Moreover, the connotation of some rhythms remains unclear. For example, the rhythm of "ten days" is often used in Huangdi's Canon of Medicine to anticipate the outcome of the disease. However, the ten-day rhythm has no support from more adequate materials except for the statement in Yinyangxiriyue Article of Spiritual Pivot that ten fingers corresponding to ten days, and the essence and biological manifestation of ten-day rhythm remain unknown.

INTERNAL ORGAN SYNDROMES AND TRADITIONAL CHINESE MEDICINE

Internal organ syndromes require a practitioner to first make a general diagnosis before treatment can commence. In this way, traditional Chinese medicine is similar to Western medicine. However, a practitioner uses different methods to make a diagnosis – taking into account the eight parameters, the vital substances, and the pernicious influences.

Once a practitioner establishes a general diagnosis, the next step is to determine which organ systems are affected. This logical procedure leads to a final diagnosis that is specific enough to enable the physician to prepare a focused treatment plan.

For example, a patient may have chronic night sweats, irritability, and thirst – general signs of yin deficiency – but the practitioner still does not know which organ system to nourish at this point. Keeping in mind the normal functions of the organs, the practitioner might find further symptoms of palpitations, insomnia, and poor memory, concluding that the yin deficiency affects mostly the heart. The treatment plan would then include an herbal formula to nourish heart yin.

It is rare when all of the classic symptoms of a typical syndrome are present. In fact, it is more common for just a few symptoms to occur, and these often arise from two or three simultaneous disease patterns. For example, a person might have chronic spleen qi deficiency with symptoms of only poor appetite and loose stools. The same person could also have liver qi stagnation with the only symptom being premenstrual syndrome once a month. If this person catches a cold on top of these underlying disorders, her symptoms would involve three separate patterns of disharmony.

Early-stage and mild versions of syndromes may have very subtle symptom patterns; these require the diagnostic skills of an experienced practitioner. It is important to remember that the functions of organs in traditional Chinese medicine may overlap those of their Western counterparts, but they also have totally unrelated functions. For this reason, it is dangerous to attempt to find a standard correspondence between the two.

For example, a chest cold might be diagnosed as a lung condition under both systems, but asthma might be a kidney condition in traditional Chinese medical diagnostics. Both medical systems stand on their own strengths, but an attempt to artificially link the two can often make them less effective. Attempting to treat the flu simply with Chinese herbs that have antiviral qualities is less effective than getting an accurate diagnosis – wind heat, for example – and using a traditional formula for that wind heat.

CHINESE MEDICINES DERIVED FROM THE HUMAN BODY

Li Shizhen's Bencao gangmu, the classic materia medica of traditional Chinese medicine (TCM), included 35 human drugs, including organs, bodily fluids, and excreta. Crude drugs derived from the human body were commonplace in the early history of medicine. Some of these TCM human drug usages are familiar from alternative medicine, such as medicinal breast milk and urine therapy. Others are uncommon, such as the "mellified man", which was a foreign nostrum allegedly prepared from the mummy of a holy man who only ate honey during his last days and whose corpse had been immersed in honey for 100 years.

Some of these Bencao gangmu human drug names use obscure classical Chinese terms. Chǐyìn "tartar; dental calculus; plaque" (52.20) uses the rare name yìn "sediment: dregs" instead of gòu "filth" in the common yágòu. Renshi "penis" (52.32) uses shì "power; circumstance" in the archaic sense of "male genitals" seen in qùshì "castrate; emasculate".

While most names of these 35 Chinese "human drugs" (translated as hair, dandruff, and earwax) are understandable, several culture-specific terms need explanation.

Li Shizhen distinguishes drugs from four types of human hair: 52.1 fàbèi "(esp. boy's) hair cut from the head", 52.2 luànfà "hair left on a comb after using it", 52.25 zīxū "facial hair", and 52.26 yīnmáo "pubic hair". Li details additional names and their corresponding pulse diagnosis acupuncture channels.

Hair from different positions is given different names: Hair on the head, called Fa (hair), pertains to Kidney Channel of Foot Lesser Yin and Stomach Channel of Foot Greater Yang. Hair in front of the ears, called Bin (temples), pertains to Sanjiao Channel of Hand Lesser Yang and Gall Bladder Channel of Foot Lesser Yang. Hair above the eyes, called Mei (eyebrow), pertains to Large Intestine Channel of Hand Greater Yang and Stomach Channel of Foot Greater Yang. Hair on the upper lip, called Zi (moustache), pertains to Large Intestine Channel of Hand Greater Yang. Hair under the chin, called Xu (beard), pertains to Gall Bladder Channel of Foot Lesser Yang and Stomach Channel of Foot Greater Yang. Hair on the cheeks, called Ran (whiskers), pertains to Gall Bladder Channel of Foot Lesser Yang.

The obscure drug 52.14 pǐshí, translated as "gall-stones" (Read), "gallstones" and described as "hard masses formed from extraordinary addiction or devotion" (Luo), combines words meaning "craving; addiction; extreme devotion; idiosyncrasy; indigestion" and "stone; rock". Li Shizhen explains, "If a person is especially devoted to a certain habit or thing, or when a person is suffering from the formation of hard masses, a strange thing will take shape." Li gives examples of similar things "formed due to congelation of a kind of essence substance": niúhuáng "ox bezoar; calculus bovis", gǒubǎo "stone in a dog's kidney/gall bladder", zhǎdá "white stone that forms between the liver and gall of livestock, used for rain prayers", and shèlìzi "śarīra; a Buddhist relic supposedly found in cremated ashes".

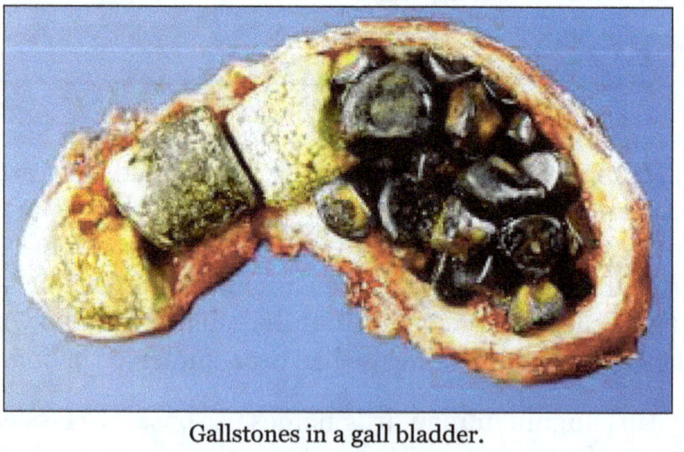

Gallstones in a gall bladder.

Medicinal 52.18 rénjīng "human semen" includes both male and female jīngyè, meaning male "seminal fluid; semen" and female "vaginal lubrication". Li Shizhen says.

> The essence substance of Ying (nutrient essence in blood) can be transformed into semen and gathered at the Mingmen (Gate of Life), which is the house of Jing (Vital Essence) and blood. When a boy is 16 years old, the volume of his semen is one sheng and six ge (over 1.5 liters). If it is well protected, it will accumulate to three sheng (nearly 5 liters). If it is not protected and is exhausted too quickly, less than a sheng of it can be retained. Without blood, semen cannot form. Semen is a treasured thing within the body and is well nourished by qi (Vital Energy). Therefore, when blood is at its full capacity, the amount of semen will be increased. When qi (Vital Energy) accumulates, semen becomes overfilled. Evil alchemists fool stupid maidens and mate with them. Then they drink the vaginal secretions of the girls. Or they blend their own semen with the menstrual blood of a maiden and eat it. This mixture is called Qiangong (lead and mercury). They consider this a treasured drug and indulge in sex excessively, eating such a foul thing. This practice will shorten their lifespans greatly.

Both 52.12 qiūshí "processed white sediment of human urine with salt" and 52.30 bāoyīshuǐ "processed fluid of human placenta" specify particular methods of iatrochemical or medical-chemical preparation.

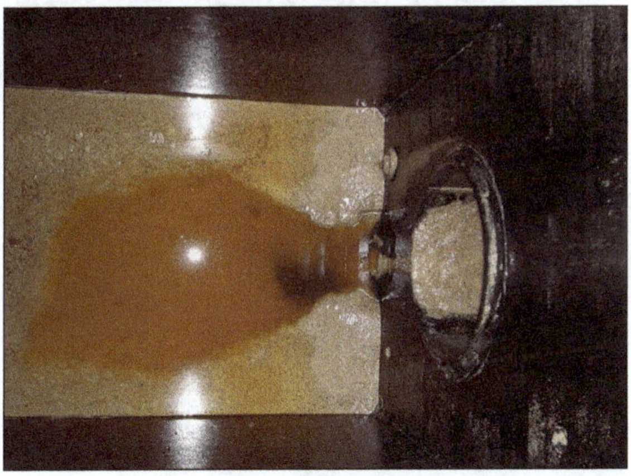

Urine precipitate in a tank collecting urine from urine diversion flush toilets in Germany.

Qiūshí (lit. "autumn mineral"), translated as "urea" (Read) and "processed white sediment of human urine with salt" (Luo), was prepared from 52.11 nibaiyin "white urinary sediment" from the urine of either Yin girls or Yang boys. The qiushi drug was called qiūbīng (lit. "autumn ice") after recrystallization, similar to boiling seawater to get salt. Li Shenzhen warns that, "Some alchemists fake the product by calcining salt in a furnace. Any substance alleged to be Qiubing should be examined carefully to make sure it is genuine." Li Shizhen outlines historical changes in the use of steroid-rich urine drugs. In ancient times, doctors used urinary precipitates to "keep the blood in motion, greatly help sexual debility, bring down heat, kill parasites, and disperse poisons; but the princes and wealthy patricians disliked using it because they considered it unhygienic. So the iatro-chemists (fangshi) began to purify the sediment, making first qiushi and later on qiubing", which licentious people used as aphrodisiacs. The Bencao gangmu lists six methods of processing qiushi through techniques including dilution, precipitation, filtration, evaporation, calcination, and sublimation.

Bāoyīshuǐ, translated as "old liquefied placenta" and "fluid of human placenta" (Luo), was traditionally processed in two ways. In north China, people bury a human placenta in the ground for 7 to 8 years, and it dissolves into a fluid that is as clean as ice. In south China, people blend human placenta with gāncǎo "Glycyrrhiza uralensis; Chinese licorice root", shēngmá "Cimicifuga simplex; bugbane", and other drugs, which they store in a bottle, and bury in the ground for 3 to 5 years. Then they dig it up and use it medicinally.

The 52.24 rénpò "Human ghost (of a hanged person)" medicine refers to Chinese hun and po soul dualism between the hun "spiritual, ethereal, yang soul" that leaves the body after death and the po "corporeal, substantive, yin soul" that remains with the corpse. Li Shizhen explains, "Renpo is found in the soil under a person who has hanged himself or herself. It resembles soft charcoal. If the Renpo is not dug out in time, it will penetrate deep into the earth where it cannot be traced." The Bencao gangmu compares a hanged person's soul with similar phenomena, "When a star descends to the earth it turns into a stone. When a tiger dies, his eyesight descends and turns into a white stone. Human blood will turn into phosphorus or jade when it drops to the ground." Li only gives one prescription, "Renpo pacifies the Heart and tranquilizes the soul and boldness. It treats convulsions, fright, and manic-depressive psychosis. Grind Renpo with water and take it by mouth."

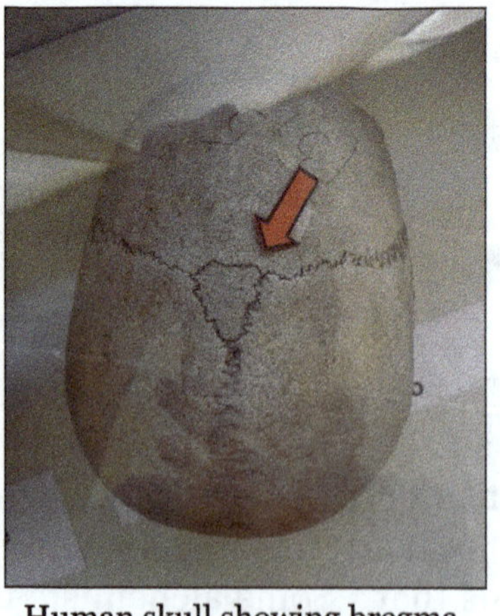

Human skull showing bregma.

52.28 Tiānlínggài "bregma; skullcap; calvaria" is translated as "human skull" (Read), "human skull top" (Luo), and "bregma" (Cooper & Sivin). In Daoist meditation and qigong breathing practices, the bregma is considered the locus of the upper dantian "elixir field". Li Shizhen says, "The skull of a human looks like a round cover. It is shaped like the sky. It is the palace of Niwan" – níwán "clay pellet" is a Chinese transcription of "nirvana". Furthermore, "It is a place where ancestral wisdom is stored.

Taoist alchemists stimulate the Li (Fire) by Kan (Water) so as to restore its condition of pure Qian (Yang). In this way, a sacred fetus will form. Then it may go out and come back in as it wishes. So the top of the skull is called Tianlinggai (meaning "cover of the Heavenly wisdom")." This shèngtāi "sacred embryo/fetus; Embryo of Sainthood" denotes achieving xian immortality through neidan "internal alchemy". Cooper & Sivin say drilling the skull in order to provide a passage is still part of the initiation ritual for members of the esoteric Shingon sect in Taiwan today.

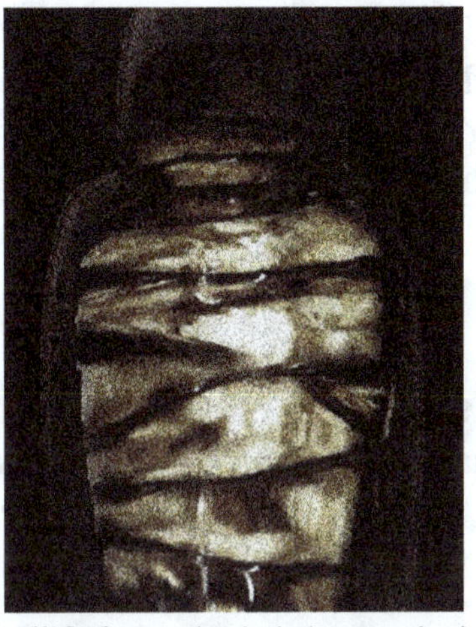

Mellified man (artistic impression).

The 52.35 mùnǎiyī "mummy; mellified man" drug was not a Chinese drug and came from Tianfangguo, which was an archaic name for "Arabia; Middle East". Li Shizhen recounts this foreign legend and expresses skepticism:

> The book Chuogeng Lu by Tao Jiucheng: It is recorded that in the Tianfang country there was an old man 70 or 80 years old was willing to sacrifice his body for the general public. So he stopped taking any food except for drinking honey daily. He washed himself repeatedly. After a month, his stools and urine all turned into honey. After his death, people in the country kept him in a stone coffin filled with honey. The date was inscribed on the stone coffin and it was buried in the ground. After 100 years, the body became a kind of honey-preserved thing that was used as a drug. When someone was suffering from an injury to his body, including bone fractures, a little of the "honey man" could be taken as a drug. It worked right away. Even in that country, this was something very precious. It was called "honey man. The above is quoted from Tao Jiucheng's book. It is not known whether this is true or not.

Among this total content of 35 entries with 287 prescriptions, 13 human drugs with 217 prescriptions first appeared in the Bencao gangmu while 22 types with 67 prescriptions came from earlier Chinese materia medica: 1 from the Eastern Han dynasty Shennong bencaojing; 5 from the Liang dynasty Mingyi bielu; 9 from the Tang dynasty Xinxiu bencao and Bencao shiyi; 8 from Song dynasty texts Da Ming rihua bencao, Kaibao bencao, Jiayou bencao, and Zhenglei bencao; and 1 other from the Ming dynasty Bencao mengquan. A few Bencao gangmu prescriptions are cited from non-medical literature, such as Zhang Hua's Bowuzhi "Record of Wide Knowledge" collection of wonders (but this magical marital formula is not found in the current reconstituted version). Prescription 52.16.5, "To keep one's wife from being jealous. Wrap a toad in the cloth the wife uses to absorb her menses and bury it five [cun] (15 cm) deep, one chi (31 cm) in front of the privy."

Since more than one-third of the human drugs were first added in Li Shizhen's time, "research into the origin of these relatively recent remedies which may reveal a new interchange of thought and practice between China and other civilizations. It may have been that the Arabs were in this matter a common source of both Chinese and European medicine."

Sample Entry

Bencao gangmu drug entries typically give the name used in the earliest materia medica reference, synonyms, explanations from earlier authors, information about preparing the drug, indications, effects, and prescriptions.

433. YIN MAO. PUBIC HAIR (M & F).

Shih-Yi: Pubic hair of the male is used for snake bite. Twelve [sic] hairs held in the mouth and sucked will keep the poison from entering the viscera.

For difficult labour, 14 hairs from the husband ashed and taken with lard in the form of a pill.

Pubic hair from the female is used to treat gonorrhea and sexual diseases. Also for swollen belly in the cow.

This "Shih-Yi" abbreviates Chen Cangqi's Bencao Shiyi "Supplement to Materia Medica". Read translates yinyangyibing (lit. "yin-yang exchange disorders") as "gonorrhea and sexual diseases", compare Luo's "febrile disease transmitted by sex" below. According to Cooper & Sivin, yinyangyi is a general name for "illnesses contracted through sexual intercourse with someone who has just recovered from them", which are diagnosed by the appearance of a yang pulse on the wrist under conditions in which a yin pulse is normally read, and vice versa.

CLAUSE 52-26 YINMAO

Human pubic hair – Bencao Shiyi (Supplement to Materia Medica by Chen Cangqi).

Indications

Chen Cangqi: Male pubic hair is a good antidote for snake bite. Hold 20 strands of pubic hair in the mouth, and swallow the juice. This will prevent the snake's toxin from entering the abdomen.

Human pubic hair is good for treating dystocia with transverse or footling presentation. Burn 14 pieces of pubic hair of the patient's husband, blend the residue with pig lard, and make into pills the size of soy beans. Swallow the pills. – Qiaijin Yaofang (Essential Prescriptions worth a Thousand Gold).

Li Shizhen: Female pubic hair is good for treating stranguria of five types and the Yinyangyi syndrome (febrile disease transmitted by sex).

Prescriptions Two prescriptions collected recently.

Prescription 52.26.1: To treat the Yinyangyi syndrome (febrile disease transmitted by sex): After a man has just recovered from a serious disease, and he has sex too soon, his scrotum will become swollen and will shrink into his abdomen. This will be accompanied by severe colic. Burn female pubic hair into ash and take it by mouth right away. Also drink water in which female genitalia have been washed. – Puji Fang

Prescription 52.26.2: To treat an ox that is dying from the effects of a distended abdomen: Wrap female pubic hair in straw and feed it to the ox.

Luo explains "As most of the "drugs" from human being are no more used medically, it seems rude to list them as drugs." Note the medical terms dystocia "A slow or difficult labor or delivery" and stranguria (i.e., strangury "A painful, frequent need to urinate, when the bladder is largely empty or with little urine production").

Moral Aspects

Reflecting the well-known Confucianist inhibition against mutilating one's body:

> The human is a different species from all the other organisms used as sources of drugs. In later times, Taoist alchemists considered that many parts of the human body should be used as drugs, such as bone, flesh, and gall. This is really very rude and inhuman. In the present category, all parts of the human body that have been used as drugs are recorded. The use of drugs from the human body that is not contrary to morality is recorded in detail. Those drugs that are cruel or foul are not recorded in detail. But all of them are listed in this category.

Li does not give prescriptions for 12 of the 35 human drugs, which he considered "cruel or foul".

Li Shizhen sharply criticized medicinal usage of bone and flesh:

> In ancient times, people thought it a benevolent deed to bury discarded human bones. Such people thought that they would be rewarded with good. But some

> alchemists collect human bones and use them as a drug with the hope of making a profit from them. Should this be done to those who save people from diseases? Even dogs do not eat the bones of dogs. Why should a human eat the bones of other humans?

Under the 52.34 human flesh entry, Li denounces two earlier pharmacopeias. Chen Cangqi's (early 8th century) Bencao Shiyi prescribes flesh as a good drug for láozhài "consumptive and infectious diseases", and Li Shizhen says, "Our bodies, skin, and hair are inherited from our parents and should be well protected. Even when parents are seriously ill, how can they bear to eat the flesh of their offspring? This is a practice followed only by stupid, foolish folk." Li Shizhen quotes Tao Jiucheng's (8th century) Chuogeng Lu, "In ancient and present-day warfare, soldiers have eaten human flesh, calling it Xiangrou (meaning "imagine it as meat") or Liangjiaoyang (meaning meat of sheep with two legs")", and comments, "This is done by bandits and thieves without human hearts. Such damned villains".

Luo's "those whose genitals are physically damaged" euphemistically translates the original metaphor cánshì "silkworm nursery; (traditional) prison where the punishment of castration was inflicted". Compare Cooper & Sivin's version, "Contemplating this story, it would seem that those 'who go down to the silkworm room' [who are administratively sentenced to castration] should not be ignorant of this method, so I append it here."

In some Bencao gangmu contexts concerning human drugs, Li Shizhen would accept the traditional theory but deny the contemporary practice. Under the human breath or qi section, Li says a "very effective" method for treating an elderly person who is suffering from cold and deficiency in the lower body is to have a boy or girl blow air through a cloth into the navel. However, he notes that contemporary "Taoist alchemists have advocated the following way of using this energy. Let a maiden breathe air into the nostrils, umbilicus, and penis of an old man. This will provide a connection between the three Dantians (the elixir fields at the upper, middle and lower regions of the body)." Li Shizhen moralistically warns, "This is a small skill practiced by alchemists. If this is not done exactly as stipulated, such practice can only bring harm to the person."

Scientific Analysis

Lu Gwei-djen and Joseph Needham, historians of science and technology in China, analyzed urinary steroid hormones in the first serious scientific study of Chinese human drugs. They researched early references to the concentrated sex hormone preparations (52.11) nibaiyin "white urinary sediment" and (52.12) qiushi "processed urinary sediment", which Li Shizhen says were respectively first recorded in the (659) Xinxiu bencao and in the Bencao mengchuan materia medica. The Chinese use of urine as a medicine, especially for impotence and other sexual disorders, has a long history. The Book of the Later Han described three Daoist fangshi "adepts; magicians" who lived in the late 2nd century; Gan Shi, Dongguo Yannian, and Feng Junda "were all expert at following the techniques of [Rong Cheng, a semi-legendary figure associated with sexual physiology] in commerce with women. They could also drink urine and sometimes used to hang upside down. They were careful and sparing of their seminal essence and (inherited) [qi], and they did not boast with great words of their powers." Based upon the Bencao gangmu list of six methods processing urine to produce qiushi, Lu & Needham conclude that from the 11th century onwards, Chinese alchemists, physicians, and iatro-chemists were successfully making quasi-empirical preparations of active substances with androgens and estrogens, a technique that modern biochemists did not develop until the early 20th century.

The physician William C. Cooper and the sinologist Nathan Sivin chose what the Chinese call rényào "human drugs" as a pilot experiment sample for pharmacologically analyzing the efficacy of drugs used in TCM. In contrast to many traditional Chinese plant, animal, and mineral pharmaceuticals with uncertain active constituents, the chemical composition of the human body and parts is well known, and "their therapeutic effectiveness, or lack of it, can be objectively, if approximately, estimated without reference to their Chinese context." They selected 8 widely used human drugs from the 37 listed in Bencao gangmu: human hair, nails, teeth, milk, blood, semen, saliva, and bone. For each substance, Cooper and Sivin first analyzed the Bencao gangmu information about drug preparation and use, and then commented on the known chemical composition of the human drug and other ingredients in the prescriptions.

Cooper & Sivin applied the criteria of clinical pharmacology to analyze the possible medicinal value of the Bencao gangmu pharmacopeia's human drug prescriptions for 66 diseases, 58 (88%) of which prescribe one or more ancillary ingredients. Fifty (76%) diseases treated would not have been relieved strictly by known properties of the prescription constituents or their combinations, and the other sixteen (24%) diseases might possibly be benefited from the human drug, another ingredient, or their synergistic combination.

These 24% conceivably beneficial human drug prescriptions can be divided into positive and possible types. First, positive specific benefits for the ailments could come from effects of three (5%) human drug prescriptions alone (all for human blood, e.g., 52.17.3 drink blood mixed with water for internal hemorrhage from wounds), two (3%) ancillary ingredients alone (52.15.11 [not breast milk but] desiccant tung oil is "miraculously effective" for calf sores). Second, uncertain or nonspecific therapeutic benefits include five human drugs (e.g., 52.6.14 powdered left-hand fingernails and rush pith form a sticky mass applied to the canthus for removing foreign bodies in the eye), three (5%) ancillary ingredients (52.6.11 pack and roast a silkworm cocoon with a man's fingernail trimmings and a boy's hair for ulcerated hemorrhoids), and three combinations of them (52.15.7 human milk and copper coins cooked in a copper vessel for trachoma could form copper sulfate, which has a mild antibacterial effect for eye infections).

The authors conclude that less than 8% of all these disorders could have been "positively cured by known pharmacological effects of the remedies cited", and raise the question of psychosomatic or social effects of human drugs in folk medicine.

Ritual Aspects

Having demonstrated that the effectiveness of most Bencao gangmu human drug prescriptions was not attributable to pharmacognosy, Cooper & Sivin examined whether the symbolic aspects of magic and ritual in Chinese folk medicine could explain why pharmacopoeias continue to list human drugs. Within their sample of 8 human drugs, prescriptions mention two dozen symbolic ritual procedures. Sympathetic magic, for example, could explain using blood to treat blood loss (52.17.3 above) and attempting to treat bone damage with bone (52.27.1). Li Shizhen quotes the Miscellaneous Morsels from Youyang:

> The book Youyang Zaju: Once a military man in Jingzhou had an injured tibia. Doctor Zhang Qizheng treated him with a kind of medicinal wine, which was taken orally. A small segment of broken bone in the wounded tibia was taken out and a kind of medicinal ointment was applied externally. The injury was cured. The patient kept the small piece of bone from his tibia under his bed. But two years later there was a recurrence. Doctor Zhang said that the bone from the tibia was cold now. He searched for the bone and found it under the man's bed. He washed the bone with hot water, wrapped it in silk fabric, and kept in a good place. After that the pain was gone. This shows the interrelationship between the bone left under the bed and the pain. How can we say a withered bone has no sense? People should be aware of this.

Prescription 52.27.4 specifies using a dead child's bone: "To treat bone fractures: Bone of infant, calcined, and muskmelon seed, stir-fried. Grind the above ingredients into powder, and take the powder by mouth with good wine. It stops the pain right away."

Demonic possession and demonic medicine are ancient Chinese beliefs. For example, the Bencao gangmu (52.28) says "bregma; skull bone" is good for treating several tuberculosis-like diseases that are supposedly caused by evil spirits. The (sometimes synonymous) names of these sicknesses are difficult to translate, as shown by the following renderings by Cooper & Sivin, Luo and Zhang & Unschuld:

- Chuánshī "cadaver vector disease", "consumptive and infectious disease", "corpse [evil] transmission".
- Shīzhù "cadaver fixation disease", "consumptive and infectious disease", "corpse attachment-illness".
- Gǔzhēng "bone-steaming disease", "consumptive disease with general debility", "bone steaming".

- Guǐ[qì]zhù, "consumptive disease of unknown cause", "demon [qi] attachment-illness".

Li Shizhen quotes Chen Cangqi's explanation that when a piece of skull is cleaned, simmered in a young boy's urine, and then buried in a pit, "This will infuse the drug with a soul". Li also quotes Yang Shiying that the shizhu disease "is caused by a ghost that hides within a person's body and does not come out. So the disease is a prolonged one. When treated with human skull top, the ghost's soul will be dispelled from the person's body and the syndrome may subside." Cooper & Sivin note that the guzheng "bone-steaming disease" or chuanshi "cadaver vector disease", "passes from one member of a family to another, sapping their strength and killing them in turn. The name comes from the patient's feeling of feverishness ("steaming") in the marrow of his bones. The syndrome as described in classic medical works corresponds on the whole to that of pulmonary tuberculosis." However, they also say that whether this demon disease really meant pulmonary tuberculosis or some other debilitating infectious disease is really not pertinent "because bone would be ineffective in the treatment of any infectious process."

Prescription 52.28.1 Tianlingaisan "Powder of human Skull Top", which is said to be "good for killing worms in a consumptive disease", mentions seeing a chuanshi. First, take "one piece of human skull top two fingers wide, simmer the drug with Tanxiang/sandalwood, then stir-fry with Su/butter. Then chant incantations." Fifteen herbal ingredients are added with the skull bone into a decoction, which will cause the patient to defecate "worms of strange shapes". Cooper & Sivin translate the chant that Luo omits, "This incantation is recited seven times in one breath: "Divine Father Thunder, Sage Mother Lightning, if you meet a cadaver vector you must control it. Quickly, quickly, as ordered by the law." This same prescription also mentions Daoistic ritual purification, "Before the drug is processed, one who prepares the drug should abstain from meat and wine and should stay in a clean, quiet room far away from the patient, so that he cannot smell it. When the drug is prepared, keep away chickens, dogs, cats and other animals, as well as sons in mourning and women. The room should be kept clear of all ugly and dirty things."

Prescription 52.28.2 is for treating guzheng "bone-steaming disease": "To treat consumptive disease with general debility and hectic fever due to Yin deficiency: Stir-fry a piece of human skull the size of a comb until it turns yellow. Then simmer it in five sheng of water until two sheng are left. Drink the decoction in three drafts. This is a drug that will cure the patient very effectively."

Two other cases of human-drug treatments for demonic medicine are sānshī "Three Corpses; demonic spirits believed to live in the human body and hasten death" and gǔdú gu poisoning; a poison produced by venomous insects; cast a black magic spirit possession over someone".

The first Bencao gangmu prescription for human nails is not from Chinese medical texts but from Daoist rituals for expelling what describe as the "Three Corpse-Worms, the chief of the "inner gods" who are to the individual microcosm what the celestial bureaucracy is to the cosmos." Prescription 52.6.1, the "Method of Beheading the Three Corpses", involves supernaturally cutting the nails in accordance with the traditional 60-day sexagenary cycle in the Chinese calendar and Chinese astrology. Luo footnotes that Daoists believe sanshi to be "a kind of spirit haunting a patient. It may also be manifested as subcutaneous nodes appearing on three portions of the body cavity."

Gudu-poisoning diseases are supposedly treatable with four human drugs: dandruff, teeth, feces, and placenta. For instance, "To treat Gudu (disease caused by noxious agents produced by various parasites), no matter whether caused by a herb, a snake, or a dung beetle: It seems as if such things enter into the throat, causing terrible pain and making the patient feel as if he is dying. Wash a Ziheche/placenta hominis/dried human placenta and cut it into slices. Dry the slices in the sun and grind them into powder. Wash down one qianbi [an ancient coin] of the powder each time with boiled water."

Modern Medicine

Present day Chinese doctors and herbalists continue to prescribe human drugs, despite their lack of proven efficacy. Cooper & Sivin note that a modern TCM pharmacognosy handbook lists 634 medicinal substances, including 5 from humans: placenta, fingernails, ashed hair, urine, and urine sediment.

Four centuries after Li Shizhen considered the bioethical and biomedical dilemmas of using human drugs, 20th-century technological and medical advances have raised new related questions of organ transplants, transplantation medicine, organ trade, tissue banks, human cloning, and the commodification of human body parts.

RELATIONSHIP BETWEEN TRADITIONAL CHINESE MEDICINE AND MODERN MEDICINE

The essence of the traditional Chinese medicine has always been the most advanced and experienced therapeutic approach in the world. It has knowledge that can impact the direction of future modern medical development; still, it is easy to find simple knowledge with mark of times and special cultures. The basic structure of traditional Chinese medicine is composed of three parts: one consistent with modern medicine, one involuntarily beyond modern medicine, and one that needs to be further evaluated. The part that is consistent with modern medicine includes consensus on several theories and concepts of traditional Chinese medicine, and usage of several treatments and prescriptions of traditional Chinese medicine including commonly used Chinese herbs. The part that is involuntarily beyond modern medicine contains several advanced theories and important concepts of traditional Chinese medicine, relatively advanced treatments, formula and modern prescriptions, leading herbs, acupuncture treatment and acupuncture anesthesia of traditional Chinese medicine that affect modern medicine and incorporates massage treatment that has been gradually acknowledged by modern therapy. The part that needs to be further evaluated consists not only the knowledge of pulse diagnosis, prescription, and herbs, but also many other aspects of traditional Chinese medicine.

The essence of traditional Chinese medicine has always been the most advanced and experienced medicine in the world. Its vast system is full of practical medical technology and proven experiences that have been gradually incorporated into modern medicine; it has knowledge that can impact the direction of future medical development, yet its knowledge is simple enough to fit changing times and varied cultures. The basic structure of traditional Chinese medicine is composed of the following three parts: the part that is consistent with modern medicine, the part that is involuntarily beyond modern medicine, and the part that needs to be further evaluated or abandoned.

The Part that is Consistent with Modern Medicine

In the 16th century, what is now known as "western medicine" was introduced to China but was not commonly used and thus had little effect. It was not until the Opium War that "western medicine" began to develop in China. Therefore, prior to that event, traditional Chinese medicine was always the leading force of medical care in China.

The key to successful medicine lies in its efficacy. A popular Chinese saying states "Excellence is from experience." The foundation of traditional Chinese medicine is based on 5,000 years of practice and experiences. With the founding of a new China in 1949, western medicine in the region also began to play a large role in medical care. As modern (westernized) medicine's impact increased, it led to the development of "integrative medicine" at the end of the 1950s. Theories, therapeutic principles, technologies, and understanding of the life sciences were elaborated, and the basic structure of traditional Chinese medicine also became clearer. Most importantly, traditional Chinese medicine began to reach a common point with modern medicine.

Consensus on Several Theories and Conceptions of Traditional Chinese Medicine

For example, "the essence of kidney" is a core concept of traditional Chinese medical theory. Studies by Shen showed that "kidney deficiency syndrome" is equivalent to the aging in modern medicine, regardless of its external performance and internal changes. Studies by Chen et al. showed that what is known as "heart qi deficiency" is associated with cardiac insufficiency in modern medicine.

Consensus on Inspection, Auscultation-Olfaction, Inquiry and Palpation Method

There are four main components of traditional Chinese medicine diagnosis. Inspection is a method to determine the medical status by visually examining the changes in appearance and the movement of the whole body or part of the body. Generally speaking, inspection includes examination of the tongue as well as the observation of a patient's external appearance, in order to recognize the internal and external manifestations of disease. Visual examination is consistent with modern medicine's emphasis on observation of a patient appearance and movement. For example, a pale lip can indicate anemia in modern medicine.

The use of auscultation-olfaction, including listening to the sounds and smelling for odors, is also consistent with modern medicine. If a patient speaks loudly and powerfully, the physician can determine that the patient is full of energy. Conversely, if a patient's voice is weak or he does not want to talk, it is most likely that the patient's diseases are caused by "deficiency." A patient's bodily odors can also reveal much about the respective illness. If a patient has a rotten apple like odor, it is likely diabetic ketoacidosis. Inquiry refers to the gathering of a thorough history and reviewing the systems. These include physical and mental feelings, life history, family history, past medical history, onset time, and the present symptoms, which are widely used both in traditional medicine and modern medicine.

Consensus on Several Treatments of Traditional Chinese Medicine

Therapeutic studies show that Chinese medicine and modern medicine have reached a consensus on the methods of diaphoresis, purging, vomiting, warming, clearing, neutralizing, eliminating, and reinforcing (eight commonly used treatments in traditional Chinese medicine). For instance, the "reinforcing method" is able to improve neuroendocrine regulatory function, enhance the body's ability to combat stress, adjust immune function, and improve the body's systemic function. Diaphoresis is able to promote perspiration and defervescence as well as play a role in reducing inflammation among other methods adopted by modern medicine.

Consensus on Several Prescriptions of Traditional Chinese Medicine and Commonly used Chinese Herbs

Several ancient herbal formulas that form consensus with modern medicine. There are many Chinese herbs either given as single drugs or as formulations that have been effective treatments for particular illnesses for thousands of years. With the development of modern medicine, the pharmacology and mechanism of action of many of these Chinese herbs have been determined, so that traditional Chinese medicine has gradually formed a consensus with modern medicine. Consensus of several commonly used herbs.

The Part ahead of Modern Medicine Involuntarily

Traditional Chinese medicine is a practical medicine built on experience. The theoretical system is built by means of an ancient plain materialist philosophy, the method of "syndrome differentiation," and the use of natural means to treat illness rather than emphasizing consistency with contemporary science and technology. Unlike modern medicine that has view that "Nature that cannot be certified cannot be conquered," keeping abreast of requirements of contemporary science, traditional Chinese medicine with the overall old and simple features involuntarily gives awareness beyond the era. The so-called "integrative medicine" is able to reveal this essence continually.

Several Advanced Theories and Important Conceptions of Traditional Chinese Medicine

In terms of medical theories and ways of thinking, traditional Chinese medicine has a significant contribution to modern medicine. For example, the theory of the "correspondence between man and universe" in traditional Chinese medicine is the unified outlook of body and environment. What are known as the "biological life" theory and the "biological clock" theory in modern medicine refers to the patterns of hormone secretion, and treating diseases according to the place of origin are all the embodiment of "correspondence between man and universe." The views of "unity of opposites" and "balance amongst dynamic forces" indicate the existence of universal laws in human life. Although these views are emphasized in modern life science, both approaches differ from traditional Chinese medicine because traditional Chinese medicine always considers these views as its guiding ideology and as fundamental law. Therefore, the cognitive degrees of Chinese medicine and western medicine in these views are of difference.

For example, studies by Shen show that "kidney deficiency" is due to neuroendocrine disturbance and preaging of the function of the hypothalamic-pituitary axis, which is consistent with the hypothesis that "the senile bell lies in hypothalamus" proposed by Everiff in the 1980s. However, the practice of traditional Chinese medicine precedes modern medicine by thousands of years. Our study found that the knowledge of "chronic disease involving kidney" in traditional Chinese medicine has a profound connotation in modern life sciences. Many diseases, such as airway inflammatory diseases, with long-term recurrence, often exacerbate the pathological changes in the anti-inflammatory system and HPA axis. Patients suffering from these are known to have significant "kidney deficiency." We summarized many theories and concepts with advanced knowledge in traditional Chinese medicine in.

Several Relatively Advanced Treatments of Traditional Chinese Medicine

"Same treatment for different diseases," one of the most important and characteristic concepts in traditional Chinese medicine reflects the spirit of "syndrome differentiation and treatment" and refers to the thought that different diseases at certain stages of development show the same pathogenesis. And therefore, the same therapeutic principles can be applied to diseases. For example, according to modern medical diagnosis, different diseases are able to be cured by "reinforcing kidney and replenishing qi" as long as they are attributed to "kidney-qi deficiency" syndrome. Modern research has shown that this concept of "same treatment for different diseases" is likely to be one of the directions of modern medicine in the future. Because some of the "walls" that exist between the diseases are not always reasonable, the reason for division is often based on anatomy, rather than etiological and pathological changes. Studies have shown that different diseases with similar syndrome often have common pathological and physiological changes. It is easier to achieve better effects by using the same prescription because different diseases may have comparable changes at the cellular, molecular, and genetic levels, and drug targets or the target groups may be similar across various diseases.

Several Relatively Advanced Formula and Modern Prescriptions

Realgar-Indigo Naturalis Formula

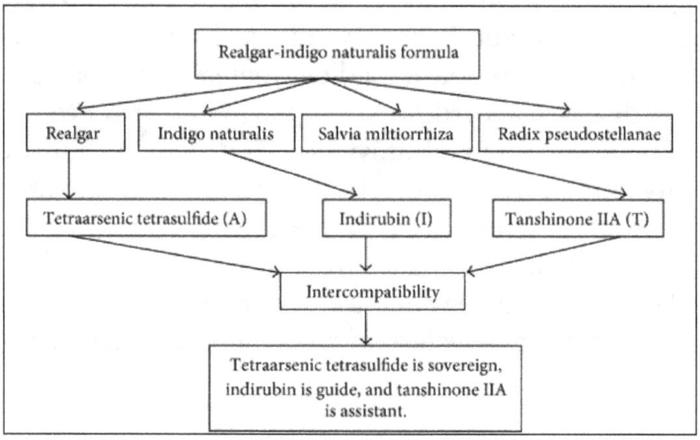

Realgar-Indigo naturalis formula.

Acute promyelocytic leukemia (APL) has a poor prognosis. In the 1980s, a famous Chinese medical expert in China, Doctor Shi-lin Huang, designed a Realgar-Indigo naturalis formula (RIF), in which, realgar, a mined ore, is the principal element and Indigo naturalis, Salvia miltiorrhiza, and Radix psudostellariae are adjuvant components to assist the effects of realgar. The main components of RIF are realgar, Indigo naturalis, and Salvia miltiorrhiza, with tetraarsenic tetrasulfide (A), indirubin (I), and tanshinone IIA (T) as major active ingredients, respectively. Multicenter clinical trials showed that a complete remission rate of 96.7% to 98% and a 5-year overall survival rate of 86.88% were achieved in APL patients receiving RIF, with moderate adverse effects such as gastrointestinal discomfort and rash. Doctor Zhu Chen clarified the molecular mechanism of the compound Huangdai tablets in the treatment of APL in 2008 from the perspective of molecular biology and biochemistry in the renowned journal Proceedings of the National Academy of Sciences of the United States of America (PNAS). The results show that As_4S_4 induces degradation of the cancer protein, thus reversing the increase in cancer cells and making them differentiate and mature. Tanshinone and indirubin promote the ubiquitination of the oncoprotein and accelerate its degradation, further promoting the differentiation and maturation of the leukemia cells and inhibiting cell cycle and proliferation of cancer cells. Animal studies also showed that the use of natural indigo after realgar substantially reduced toxicity. These reflect the concepts of typical "minister" (the place inferior to "monarch" drug) and "assistant" (the place inferior to "minister" drug) effect. Tanshinone and indirubin increase the production of channel proteins that deliver As4S4, which significantly increase the concentration of As4S4 in leukemia cells, improving its efficacy. Both tanshinone and indirubin play the role of "guide" (the place inferior to "assistant" drug). The compound Huangdai has a synergistic effect with the other components greater than its three individual components by the joint application of each component

Airway Stabilizer Solution

The airway stabilizer solution created by Doctor Jing-cheng Dong is based on Xiao Qing Long Tang (Little Dragon Decoction) and Ding Chuan Tang (Anti-asthmatic Decoction), composed of ligusticum wallichii, ginkgo biloba, skullcap, Asarum, ginger, almonds, earthworm, rehmannia, and magnolia. It is effective in the clinical treatment of bronchial asthma and variability of cough. The various components and the basis for its efficacy are rooted in traditional Chinese medical theory, and the composition of the drug may be the main material basis for its efficacy.

Table: Components and ingredients of the airway stabilizer solution.

Name	Herb	Ingredient
Airway stabilizer solution	Ephedra	Ephedrine and other minor components
	Ligusticum wallichii	Tetramethylpyrazine
	Ginkgo biloba	Ginkgolide
	Scutellaria	Baicalin
	Asarum	Racemic go A black alkali
	Ginger ale	Ginger oil glycosides
	Almonds	Amygdalin
	Earthworm	Earthworms antipyretic
	Rehmannia	Habitat catalpol
	Magnolia	Volatile oil

Several Leading Herbs

The study of Chinese medicine is driven in part by the development of modern pharmacology. For instance, Artemisia annua was recorded in the "Handbook of Prescriptions for Emergency" (written by Hong Ge in Eastern Jin Dynasty) as a drug used to treat malaria. Modern research has shown that it has an antimalarial active ingredient (the peroxide group of sesquiterpene lactone) consisting of only 3 elements, carbon, hydrogen, and oxygen. It is a completely different novel compound compared to known antimalarial drug structures. This finding overturned the judgment of experts who insisted that the structure of the antimalarial drugs must have a nitrogen-containing heterocyclic ring. It helps provide a direction for the design and synthesis of new drugs. In addition, ginseng, skullcap, astragalus, epimedium, and other herbs were also each shown to have a unique effect.

Acupuncture Treatment and Acupuncture Anesthesia that Affect Modern Medicine

Those who practice acupuncture approach the treatment by looking at pathology in the whole body. According to different body conditions, varied acupoints and manipulations are selected. The selection influences multiple targets and many diseases and stimulates the body to treat diseases, affecting the pathological process and improving physique.

This adjustment is accomplished by the integration of the central nervous system, including cortex recombination, neural plasticity, and release of various neurotransmitters and hormones. The basis of acupuncture may be in changes in gene expression.

Acupuncture anesthesia is a method used to prevent surgical pain and relieve physiological dysfunction. It is suitable for those who are allergic to narcotic drugs. Since 1958, Shanghai No. 1 People's Hospital used it instead of narcotic drugs to perform tonsillectomies. Since then, acupuncture anesthesia has been passed from general usage to selected application. According to its clinical effect and scientific evaluation, acupuncture anesthesia is effectively used in thyroid surgery, surgery of posterior cranial fossa, craniocerebral operation, anterior cervical surgery, pulmonary resection, caesarean section, tubal ligation, and tooth extraction. It is also used in some surgeries with uncertain results like hysterectomy, caldwell-luc operation, subtotal gastrectomy, and strabismus surgery. It has not proved to provide effective anesthesia in limb surgery and perineal surgery.

The basis of acupuncture anesthesia is the adjustment to inhibit large pain pathways by the negative reflection of spinal pain. The acupuncture signal and the pain signal from the pain region transmit impulses into the brain. Acupuncture stimulates the antipain material to reduce the pain. Endogenous opioids participate in this process due to the increased release of opioids. Several neurotransmitters are related to acupuncture anesthesia, and some relatively central cerebral nuclei were found. CCK-8 has the negative-reflection-to-opioid effect, which is the vital factor of acupuncture and morphine. The effect of electric acupuncture depends on the balance of central opioid and CCK-8. The acupuncture signals can be reflected on some regional area of the brain to deal with the injury stimulations, which might be the physical basis of acupuncture anesthesia. Different frequencies of electric acupuncture differentiate the pain-relieving effects, which may be related to the specific expression of central genes. Two Hz electric acupuncture is widely used in the brain treatment, while 100 Hz has a narrow extension in the brain treatment. Psychological factors are not the deciding factors for success, but they are also quite important.

Massage Treatment that is Gradually Acknowledged by Modern Medicines

Massage treatment utilizes the particular skills with hands or limbs to practice manipulation on the surface of the body. Therefore, it has the direct effect of activating blood and dispersing stagnation, smoothing tendons, and improving malformation. On the other hand, massage reflectively influences the neuro and body fluid by acupoint-meridian-viscera network. Clinical researches show that appropriate manipulations can result in improvement of outcomes .

Modern research studies show that massage can promote blood and lymph circulation, increase metabolism, and assist the repair of soft tissue injury . The diastolic function of the heart improves, and arteriole function improves as well after massage. The total cell count increases, while lung function improves. The content of catecholamines in plasma decreases so that the autonomic nervous system is inhibited, which can cause a reduction in pain . Massage can effectively increase digestion in the stomach, adjust the secretion of stomach fluid, and release the spasm of smooth muscle . When ST36 and BL23 are manipulated, the function of periphery blood T lymphocyte elevates. Rubbing manipulation, embrocation, and kneading manipulation could increase the elasticity and glossiness of skin.

In short, skilled massage manipulation can effectively prevent diseases by the combination of static strength and motive force in a localized point or throughout the entire body.

Some Parts that need to be Newly Recognized or Abandoned

In the system of human science, including medical science, concepts change from new to old, and ideas become theories and facts. All the concepts and rules indicate the stability. However, this kind of stability is conditional, partial, and relative, while instability is absolute and unconditional. Any scientific systems should confess their demerits and rectify them so as to generate new concepts, methods, and theory. Meanwhile, the initial phase of modern medicine and traditional Chinese medicine were founded in specific cultures and eras. So TCM theory should be divided into two parts, one of which needs to be promoted, the other of which need to be abandoned. Integrative medicine is an important way to achieve this.

About Palpation

“Cunkou pulse” should be newly recognized. It belongs to the “Lung Meridian of Hand-Taiyin.” “Classic of Questioning” (written by Qui Bian in the Warring StatesPeriod) put forward that “Cunkou pulse” can detect diseases of the whole body. “Lung” controls whole meridians, is the master of “qi”, and is the origin of “qi” and “blood.” Therefore, it can reflect all the changes of viscera, meridians and “qi-blood” to diagnose diseases. “The Internal Canon of Medicine” (written in Huang in the Warring States period) pointed out that meridians include meridians and collaterals, not vessels. The pulse we palpate originates from the heart, which beats. The meridian cannot beat, so it should not be able to be palpated. The pulse is only one kind of syndrome. Not all diseases can be presented by the pulse. Therefore, palpation is part of signs, but one should be careful when palpation is the only examination method.

About Formula Prescription

Although formulary prescriptions are beneficial in medicine, they still have some demerits. It is hard to distinguish the "assistant" and the "guide" in some prescriptions, and therefore, it is necessary to conduct further research. "Compendium of Materia Medica" (written by Si-miao Sun in the Ming Dynasty) has lots of prescription to treat sterility. If a sterile female drank a cup of rain water in the spring, she would become fertile. If a sterile female stole a lamp from a rich person's bed, she would also become fertile. Even broom, dishwater, ashes on widow's bed, the wood in toilet, the trees fired by thunder, and the rope hung by itself were thought to treat diseases.

WAYS TO GLOBALIZE TRADITIONAL CHINESE MEDICINE

Nowadays, medicine is no longer for clinical diseases only. The paradigm of medicine has changed from disease to healthcare. The scope of medicine includes uses for disease treatment (therapeutic medicine), disease prevention (preventative medicine), life quality enhancement of patients and healthy individuals (functional medicine), and for improving the use of other medicines (accessory medicine).

The current paradigm of mainstream pharmaceutical discovery uses a reductionist approach to identify a target associated with disease or a single compound that can regulate a given target associated with a disease. Such compounds are expected to have potency and selectivity for the treatment of the disease targeted.

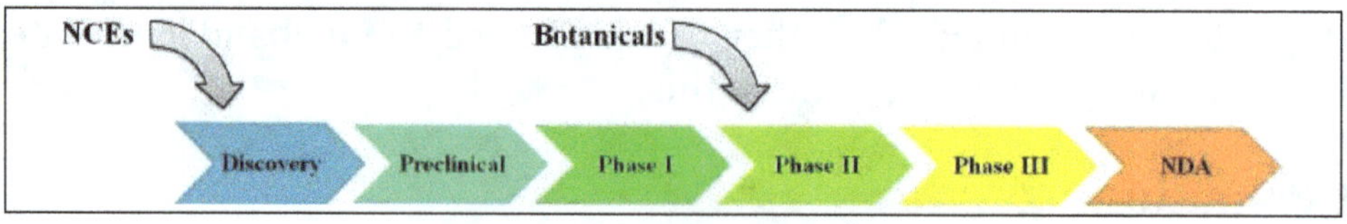

FDA Pathway for Botanical Drugs.

There are several challenges to the current mainstream drug discovery approach. A given disease can be caused by multiple reasons; therefore, it will be difficult to find one chemical with a defined target related to a specific disease, because the overall medicine helped treat a majority of the patients and prevented a majority from contracting the disease. Many potent drugs for the treatment or prevention of chronic diseases may require long-term use, and delayed toxicity may occur.

A new pharmaceutical industry, polychemical in nature, based on historical information from each geographical area, and with clinical evidence-based and consistent preparation, could be a focal point of economic development in each geographical area. Therefore, a new paradigm for future medicine is a multiple-target and polychemical medicine instead of a one-chemical medicine with a system-biology approach in mind. There are two approaches to polychemical medicine: conventional "step by step" and revisiting history as the basis of reinventing medicine.

Figure indicates the FDA pathway for botanical drugs. Botanical products with a history of safe use may start efficacy studies at Phase 2 clinical trials without preclinical requirements. Actual new drug application (NDA) requirements are identical to those of new chemical entities (NCEs), except that the combination product rule is waived; therefore, it is not necessary to study the individual active ingredients. The FDA has defined special policies for meeting chemistry, manufacturing, and control requirements; and as you might expect, this is technically quite challenging. The drug sponsor has considerable flexibility over when the required toxicology and human safety studies are conducted; therefore, development programs may be compressed with a parallel execution of toxicity, safety, and efficacy studies, or reversed as compared to NCEs with safety and toxicity studies following efficacy studies. In PhytoCeutica's view, the pathway has opened up a large pool of previously untapped drug candidates, many of which have both clinical and market validation, enabling accelerated development with a lower risk of attrition. PhytoCeutica's focus is on acute disease markets where existing therapies do not meet patients' needs.

Unique Features of Traditional Chinese Medicine

Many traditional medicines took a "holistic approach," which is just becoming an important area of medical research today. Some of these traditional medicines have claimed to meet those unmet clinical needs. Chinese herbal medicine takes a holistic approach, and is an early form of "system biology"-based "integrated medicine." Chinese medicine is prescribed on an individual basis to optimize its usage (Lu et al., 2011). It is "individualized medicine." Chinese herbal medicine has multiple medical claims for the treatment of complicated diseases, multiple symptoms, disease prevention, and life quality improvement. Chinese herbal medicine also has many chemicals that could target multiple sites, or act on a single site additively or synergistically through direct or indirect interaction (Konkimalla and Efferth, 2008). Chinese herbal medicine could meet some of the current unmet medical needs. It has its own concept, and can serve as the basis for developing future medicine.

Approaches for Advancing Traditional Chinese Medicine

The approaches for advancing traditional Chinese medicine are described in Figure.

The basic regulatory requirements for modern drugs enforce consistency of preparation, evidence-based clinical efficacy, safety, certain knowledge of a drug's action, sites of actions, active ingredients, and interactions with other drugs.

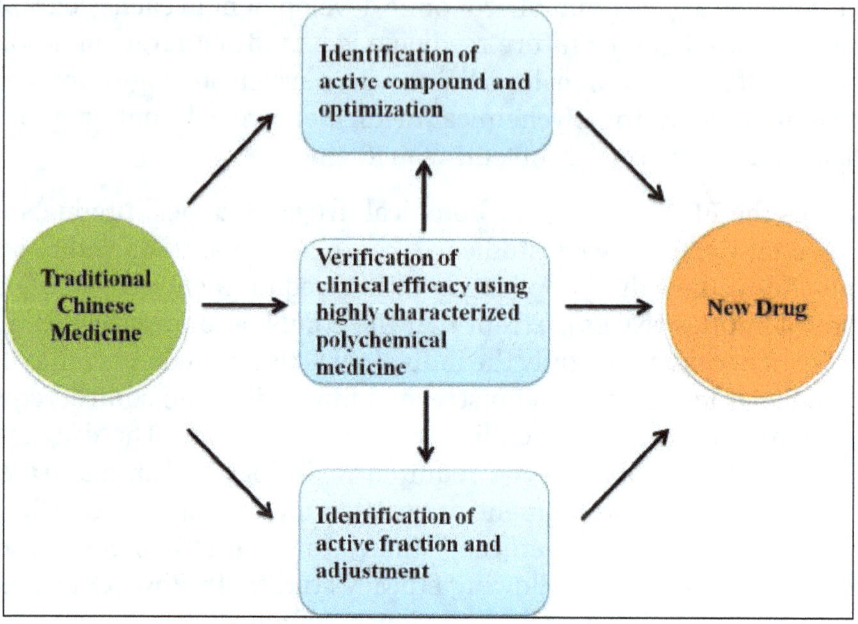

Approaches for advancing traditional Chinese medicine.

As mentioned above, the approval of Chinese herbal medicine must ensure that a consistent preparation of clinical trial material should work. Therefore, the manner in which consistent preparations of herbal medicine can be made is important. We have to identify herbs using microscopic/morphological analysis, gene sequence analysis, and chemical analysis in vitro (solution state) and in situ (solid state). We also can use Good Agricultural Practices (GAP) and Good Manufacturing Practices (GMP) to guarantee the quality of herb. Botanical/herbal medicine quality control in GAP is consistent with the use of raw herbal ingredients. GAP monitors botanical identification, collection, post-harvest processing, and agriculture contaminants, including heavy metals, pesticides, fungicides, herbicides, bacteria, plant, and fungal contaminants.

Chinese herbal medicines are mixture medicines; therefore, the quality control for complex mixtures is very important. A novel approach is required; we can use multiple parameters and inclusive Comprehensive Quality Control Measures. Moreover, there are two tiered approaches to botanical quality control (QC). Tier 1 is the fingerprint analysis, which includes global and relative quantitation by chemical fingerprint, bioresponse fingerprint, and informatics/data mining technologies. Tier 2 is the simplified analysis, which includes the specific and absolute quantitation, such as chemicals relevant to the pharmacological activity, genomic pathways, and a biological analysis relevant to the pharmacological activity, including the impact on the targeted enzyme/receptor.

Clinical trials of traditional Chinese medicine must ensure that a consistent preparation of clinical trial material is possible to produce. Double blind and placebo design is preferable in clinical trials. Other alternative designs could be taken into consideration, such as a clear clinical endpoint that is acceptable worldwide and regulations for carefully monitoring efficacy and toxicity. Statistical consideration is also critical in the drug design.

The basic study of herbal medicine includes rigorous preclinical and clinical studies, multiplex analysis, and a systems biology approach, which is driven by information and data mining.

Discoveries using the approaches outlined above for herbal medicine could facilitate the single-targeted orientation approach in Western Medicine.

Collaboration is Highly Required

The evolution of medicine is not only a responsibility for scientists but also for the botanical drug industry. The botanical drug industry should heed the following responsibilities: evidence-based therapeutic claims, high-level Quality Control, full documentation of agricultural sourcing, full use of standard operating procedures, attention to drug-botanical drug interactions, and research focuses on the mechanism of action and the identification of active phytochemicals.

The outcome of developing such a polychemical and herb-based industry will provide high-quality products based on traditional healthcare uses, decrease the cost of healthcare, provide new scientific information to advance future medicine, stimulate value-added agricultural development, and provide economic development with a regional flavor.

To globalize Chinese herbal medicine, collaboration is critical (figure). Close collaboration among academia, industry, and government is important. Given the limitation of resources (human, technological, and financial), international collaboration is critical for this advancement.

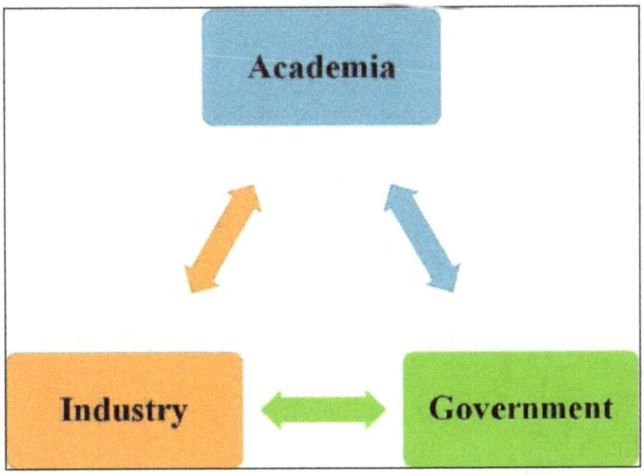

Collaboration needed to globalize Chinese and herbal medicine.

Therefore, the global, non-profit, non-discriminatory, and non-political organization Consortium for Globalization of Chinese Medicine (CGCM) was established in December 2003. The mission of CGCM is to advance the field of Chinese Herbal Medicine to benefit humankind through joint efforts with academics, industries, and regulatory agencies worldwide in the spirit of contributions and sharing.

Globalizing Chinese Medicine

In order to globalize Chinese herbal medicine, we need more scientific evidence. Figure describes the evolution of medicines.

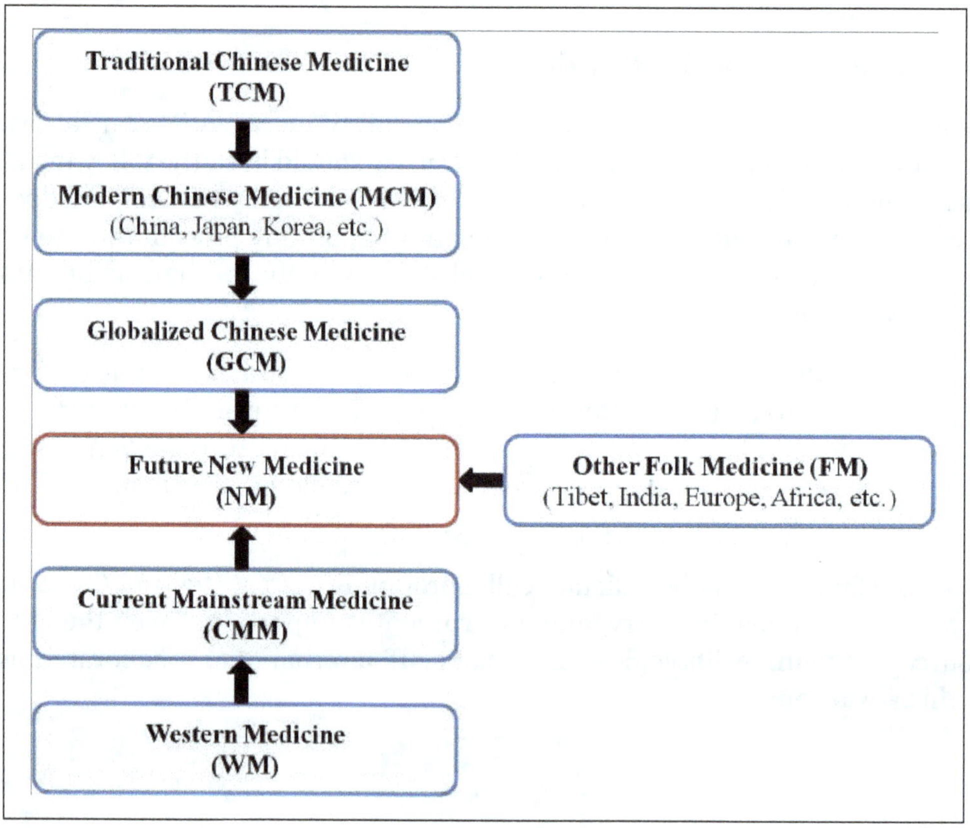

The evolution of medicine.

Chinese herbal medicine is a historical medicine with many experience-based claims; however, its defects are not very evidence-based. Therefore, the first step is to convert experience-based claims to evidence-based claims. The use of Chinese herbal medicine is based on the experiences of the doctor; and the doctor can adjust the components of the prescription through her or his own experience. Therefore, Chinese herbal medicine should add more objective quality control to prescriptions. Further, the preparation of Chinese herbal medicine involves many procedures. Some Chinese herbs require complicated processing procedures to become Chinese herbal medicine. All these requirements indicate that Chinese herbal medicine is not a friendly system for general use. Because Chinese herbal medicine formulas usually contain more than one component and the components are modulated by doctors' experiences, the practice differs from Western medicine. Chinese herbal medicine is based on a holistic approach; there is not enough scientific evidence to demonstrate safe dosage of Chinese herbs. Hence, Chinese medicines need more short-term and long-term clinical trials to understand the dosage safety of Chinese herbal medicine. If Chinese herbal medicine can overcome the defects mentioned above, it could become a mainstream medicine or a strong support for mainstream medicine. Chinese herbal medicine's interactions with mainstream medicine also need to be estimated, such as whether it collaborates in a good or bad way. Moreover, Chinese herbal medicine could use modern scientific technology to deduce its quality control, informatics, clinical uses, herbal resources, molecular mechanisms and active compounds, intellectual properties, education benefits, and industrial liaisons. We should encourage Chinese herbal medicine to become evidence-base medicine. If we could identify the resources, molecular mechanisms, etc. of Chinese herbal medicine, it could be a resource for new medicine. Overall, collaboration is a crucial point for Chinese herbal medicine; it could instigate a further evolution of medicine.

References

- What-is-tcm: tcmworld.org, Retrieved 4 June, 2020
- Traditional-chinese-medicine-what-you-need-to-know-88936: verywellhealth.com, Retrieved 26 August, 2020
- Vitamins-minerals: agelessherbs.com, Retrieved 1 April, 2020
- "deer penis loses favor as china's olympians fear drug testers". Bloomberg. March 23, 2008. Retrieved june 23, 2010
- Chinese medical herbology and pharmacology, john chen and tina chen, art of medicine press, isbn 0-9740635-0-9
- Traditional-chinese-medicine-internal-organ-syndromes, chinese, natural-medicine, wellness: howstuffworks.com, Retrieved 5 April, 2020

The Body in Traditional Chinese Medicine

CHAPTER 2

Traditional Chinese medicine believes in the circulation of the body's vital energy through channels known as meridians that are connected to body organs and functions. It divides the body into five fundamental substances - Qi, Xue, Jin ye, Zang-fu and Jing Luo. The chapter closely examines the model of body in traditional Chinese medicine to provide an extensive understanding of the subject.

QI OR VITAL ENERGY

The ancient Chinese people believed qi was the most fundamental entity making up the world. They thought everything in the universe resulted from the movement and change of qi. The Chinese character for "qi" is the same word used for air or gas, and it is thought to have the same properties as these substances. Qi can be interpreted as the "life energy" or "life force," which flows within us. Sometimes, it is known as the "vital energy" of the body.

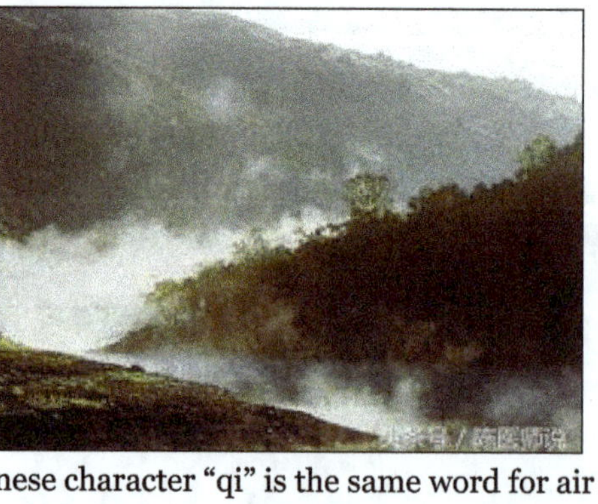

The Chinese character "qi" is the same word for air or gas.

In TCM theory, qi is the vital substance constituting the human body. It also refers to the physiological functions of organs and meridians. In fact, it may be difficult to find one equivalent English word or phrase that completely describes the nature of qi. Most often, qi is best defined according to its functions and properties.

Human qi comes from two main sources. The first source of qi is inherited from our parents at conception. It is known as the "innate vital substance". The second source is derived from essential substances in nature such as the air we breathe, food and water. Both the inherited and the acquired vital energies are further processed and transformed by the organs.

The kidney first sends the innate vital substance upwards where it combines with food essence derived from the spleen. It further mixes with the fresh air from the lungs where it finally forms into qi of the body.

By understanding how qi is formed, TCM has identified two important factors necessary for maintaining health. By eating a healthy diet and breathing fresh air, the body extracts their most valuable essences and uses them to help form the vital energy. Following these simple principles are the first steps towards creating a healthy balance in the body.

Functions of Qi

Promoting Function of Qi

Just as wind (highly active air) provides energy to push the sails of a boat or turn the turbine of a windmill, qi provides the active, vital energy necessary for the growth and development of the human body and to perform the physiological functions of the organs, meridians and tissues. In addition, qi promotes the formation and circulation of blood and supports the metabolism of body fluid. If there is a deficiency of qi, its promoting functions are weakened. As a result, growth and development can be affected or delayed, the organs and meridians cannot function properly and blood formation is hampered, leading to a series of health problems.

Warming Function

In a gaseous state, air contains more kinetic heat energy than in its liquid state. Like air, qi also contains heat energy for the body. Being a heat source, qi warms the body and keeps it at a constant temperature so normal physiological functions can take place. Deficiency of qi can lead to a lowered body temperature, intolerance of cold and cold hands and feet.

Dcfcnding Function

In TCM, one of the main causes of disease is the invasion of "Evils"."Evils" are environmental factors that lead to illness. They are classified as wind, summer heat, dampness, dryness, cold and fire. By resisting the entry of ' illness evils" into the body, qi defends against their attack and maintains healthy physiological functions. In western terms, this qi defending function acts like the immune system.

Consolidation and Retention Function

Qi consolidates and retains the body's substances and organs by holding everything in its proper place. First, qi keeps the blood flowing within the vessels and prevents it leaking out into the tissues. Secondly, qi controls and adjusts the secretion and excretion of sweat, urine and saliva, and keeps body fluids from escaping the body. Thirdly, qi consolidates and stores sperm to prevent premature ejaculation. Lastly, qi consolidates the organs and stops them from descending into a position where they cannot function properly. If qi is deficient, the consolidating function is weakened, leading to various kinds of health problems such as haemorrhage; frequent urination, premature ejaculation and stomach or kidney prolapses (where the organ sinks).

The promoting and consolidating functions work in a complementary manner. For example, qi promotes blood circulation and the distribution of body fluids, but it also controls and adjusts the secretion of fluid substances. The balance between these two functions is essential for maintaining a healthy blood circulation and water metabolism.

Transforming Functions

Qi also possesses vaporization or " transformation" functions, which are important for the metabolism of fundamental substances. As suggested by these words, qi may "vaporize" substances in the body and transform them into essence or vital energy. For example, certain actions of qi allow food to be changed into food essence, which is in turn transformed into different types of qi and blood. Indigestible food and waste are also transformed by qi into urine and stools for excretion.

Movement of Qi

The four directions of qi movement are up, down, outward and inward. These movements are so important that once qi can no longer travel in these directions, life will come to an end.

Each organ has different specialized movements. For example, spleen qi ascends the pure part of digested food from the stomach for transformation into nutritional essence. Stomach qi, on the other hand, pushes food downwards in order to remove its impurities. Some organs, like the lungs, perform movements in all four directions. Lung qi moves in and out during breathing. However, when disseminating nutritional essence to the body, lung qi ascends and then descends when liquefying waste to be sent to the kidneys.

The different movements of qi work in a coordinated manner to maintain a harmonious balance. The ascending balances the descending movement while the outward balances the inward movement. Balanced movement is important for promoting the physiological functions of different tissues, organs and meridians. Disharmonious movement of qi leads to health problems. For example, insufficient downward movement of lung qi causes a cough. When stomach qi cannot descend nausea and vomiting occurs.

Types of Qi

Qi is further classified according to its type. The four types are inborn qi, pectoral qi, nutritive qi and protective qi.

Inborn Qi

Inborn qi is the most original, essential and vital type found in the human body. It possesses prenatal and congenital properties. After conception, "congenital essence" (an essential vital substance inherited from parents) is stored in the kidney, the place from which inborn qi originates. Inborn qi is further nourished by "acquired essence" (food essence derived from digestion) of the spleen and stomach. After this process is complete, inborn qi is ready to travel to the entire body to exert its effects. Starting from the portion between the two kidneys, known as the "vital gate", the qi moves through the triple burner and circulates through the organs, muscles, skin and meridians providing the power source for all of life's activities.

Pectoral Qi

Pectoral qi is stored in the chest. It is formed by combining fresh air inhaled by the lungs and food essence derived from the spleen and the stomach. Because pectoral qi concentrates in the chest, it can penetrate the blood vessels of the heart and lungs and move outward during expiration and inward during inspiration. By flowing through the respiratory tract, pectoral qi supports the breathing function of the lungs and affects how loud the voice can be. Its ability to flow through the blood vessels and the heart is important in regulating the heartbeat and supporting the circulation of other types of qi and blood. Pectoral qi also plays a role in keeping the body warm and influences the activities of the limbs.

Nutritive Qi

Nutritive qi, as its name suggests, supplies nourishment to the body. It mainly circulates through the blood vessels with the blood. Sometimes this combination of nutritive qi and blood is referred to collectively as "nutritive blood". Nutritive qi mainly comes from food essence derived by the spleen and stomach's transformation and transportation properties. Starting from the middle burner, nutritive qi goes to the lungs where it enters the main circulation. Nutritive qi has yin properties so it can form into materials needed by other parts of the body. For example, its close relationship with blood allows it to provide some of the necessary substances needed to produce new blood. Nutritive qi also provides the needed nutrients to support the physiological functions of the organs.

Protective Qi

Protective qi protects against evils. As previously mentioned, evils are environmental factors that lead to illness. In western terms, protective qi functions like the immune system, which helps prevent disease from occurring or spreading. Unlike nutritive qi, protective qi has yang properties, because it has more functional characteristics.

Protective qi also comes from the food essence derived by the spleen and stomach. It moves outside the blood vessels and circulates in different areas from nutritive qi.

Internally, it will be distributed to the diaphragm and scattered around the chest and abdominal cavities. Externally, it moves between the skin and muscles providing protection. Protective qi not only guards against illness and disease but also regulates the sweat glands and pores and provides nourishment for the skin, hair and muscles.

Although nutritive and protective qi share the same origin, their flow directions, as previously described, are opposite to one another. By balancing their nutritive (yin) and protective (yang) functions, healthy sweating, temperature control and defence functions are maintained.

XUE OR BLOOD

XUE, or Blood, mainiy composed of the nutrient qi and body fluid, circulates inside the vessels. It is red in color and sticky in texture. Blood functions to nourish and moisten the body. It is vital to the maintenance of life.

The Production of Blood

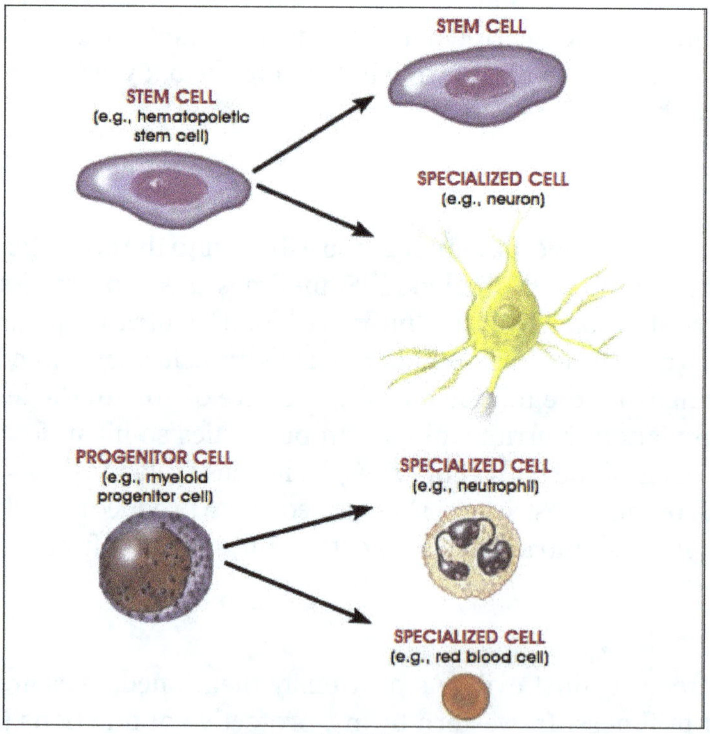

Origin of the blood cell.

The basic substance for producing blood is essence, including the congenital essence (kidney-essence) and the acquired essence (food nutrients). The congenital essence is prerequisite to the production of blood. Only when the acquired essence has combined with the congenital essence can blood be produced. Thus deficiency of kidney-essence will make it difficult to produce blood. However, the congenital essence is already fixed after birth. In this case the acquired essence plays a key role in the production of blood. For this reason the functions of the spleen and stomach are key to the production of blood. If the spleen and the stomach are normal in functions, they can absorb sufficient food nutrients to produce blood. If the spleen and stomach are weak in absorbing food nutrients, the production of blood is inevitably reduced.

The transformation of the essence into blood is in fact a process of qi-transformation. The organs involved in such a process are the heart and the lung. The function of the heart in the process of blood production is called "reddening", because the heart pertains to fire in the five elements and red in the five colors. With the action of heart-fire blood becomes red. The lung participates in the production of the nutrient qi by inhaling fresh air from the outside. The nutrient qi is an important component of blood. So the functions of the lung directly influence the production of blood. Besides, the liver regulates qi activity and influences qi-transformation in the whole body with its dredging and dispersing functions, also exerting certain effect on the production of blood.

Physiological Functions of Blood

The physiological functions of blood are to nourish and moisten the body as described in Nanjing. Since blood contains the nutrient qi, it can nourish all the organs in the body. Through the meridians, blood transports nutrient substances to all parts of the body to nourish the five zang-organs, the six fu-organs, the five constituents, the five sensory organs and the nine orifices. It should be noted that blood is also the important material base for mental activities. If blood is sufficient, there will be sufficient vitality; if blood is deficient, there will be dispiritedness; if blood is in disturbance, there will be mental disorder. Since blood contains fluid, it can moisten the viscera and the body. When the fluid flows out of the vessels, it moistens the orifices and lubricate the joints.

Besides, blood also transports the turbid qi. When the turbid qi is transported to the lung, it is excreted from respiration. When it is transported to the kidney, it is discharged from urination. When it is transported to the superficies, it is excreted from sweating.

Circulation of Blood

The vessels in the whole body form a relatively close circulatory system for blood circulation. Such a system is known as blood vessels in TCM (Traditional Chinese Medicine) included in the concept of meridians and vessels. The minute capillaries are called blood collaterals.

Blood is propelled by the heart to circulate in the vessels. In fact the heart is the center of the blood circulatory system. In structure, the heart is connected with the vessels.

That is why the heart can propel blood to circulate in the vessels. Since the circulation of blood is a circulatory process, the directions of blood circulation is either centrifugal or axopetal. The former means that the blood is propelled by heart-qi to flow out from the heart to the whole body through large vessels into large collaterals and fine capillaries. In such a way blood enters the internal organs to nourish and moisten the body. The latter means that blood accumulates from the fine capillaries to the large collaterals and the vessels into the heart under the propelling action of the heart.

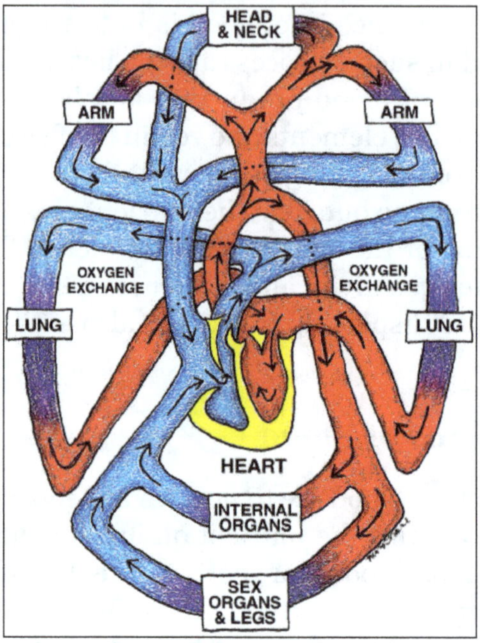

Round trip for your blood.

Apart from the heart, other internal organs are also involved in the circulation of blood, including the lung, the spleen and the liver. Structurally the lung is connected with all the vessels in the body, known as "the lung facing all the vessels". With the association with the vessels, the lung distributes nutrient substances, like the pectoral qi, to the whole body and accumulates qi and blood from the whole body to assist the heart to propel blood circulation. The spleen commands blood, making the vessels compact, directing blood to circulate normally in the vessels and preventing it from flowing out of the vessels. The liver stores blood and regulates the volume of blood. Besides, the liver also governs dredging and dispersing, thus smoothing the activity of qi to promote blood circulation.

The factor that directly acts on blood circulation is qi. For example, heart-qi propels blood to circulate; lung-qi assists the heart to propel blood circulation; spleen-qi commands blood; and liver-qi regulates the circulation of blood by dredging and dispersing qi. If heart-qi is insufficient, blood will become too weak to circulate; if lung-qi is insufficient, there will be no opportunity for blood to disperse; if spleen-qi is insufficient, it will be difficult for the spleen to command blood; if liver-qi fails to dredge, it will lead to stagnation of qi and stasis of blood. Besides, visceral yang also plays an important role in the circulation of blood. For example, deficiency of yang will inevitably cause deficiency of qi, making it difficult for blood to circulate; deficiency of yin will bring on cold and exuberant cold will coagulate blood.

Other factors that may affect blood circulation are the state of the vessels and the changes of cold and heat. Generally speaking, phlegm, dampness, blood stasis, swelling and nodules can block or compress the vessels and obstruct blood circulation. Blood is characterized by preference for warmth and aversion to cold. So excessive cold slows down the circulation of blood or even causes blood stasis; excessive heat accelerates blood circulation and even leads to bleeding in severe cases.

JIN YE OR FLUID

The word "Jin" means anything liquid or fluid. The word "Ye" means fluids of living organisms. Jin Ye = Organic Fluids.

Jin

These fluids are clear, light, thin and watery, and circulate in the exterior of the body (skin and muscles) with the Wei Qi. Under control of the Lungs, which disseminate them to the skin and of the Upper Burner, which controls their transformation and movement. Functions:

- To moisten and partly to nourish skin and muscles. (exuded as sweat, but also manifests as tears, saliva.
- To form a compound of Blood (thin out the Blood and prevent its stasis).

Ye

These are the more turbid, dense, and heavy fluids, and they circulate in the interior of the body with the Ying (Nutritive) Qi. Move relatively slowly.

Under control of (transformed by) Spleen and Kidneys, moved and excreted by Middle and Lower Burner. Functions:

- To moisten the joints, spine, brain, bone marrow.
- Lubricate the "orifices of the sense organs" i.e. eyes, ears, nose and mouth.

Body Fluids originate from food and drink.

They enter the body via the Stomach, which is said to be the origin of fluids.

The Fluids are transformed and separated into "pure" and "impure" (turbid) parts several times. Intricate series of purification processes. Pure body fluids are raised upward to the Lungs for distribution to the exterior. Impure fluids flow downward, finally excreted via the bladder.

Relationship with the Internal Organs (Zang Fu)

Stomach

The origin of fluids. Fluids first enter the Stomach where they are transformed and separated into pure and impure. Pure part goes to Spleen, impure part goes to Small Intestine and further separation. Stomach said to be "source" of body fluids.

Spleen

Very important in relation to physiology and pathology of Body Fluids. Controls the direction of flow of Fluids: pure parts upward and impure parts downward at all stages of the transformation process. The Spleen is treated in any kind of disorder of the Body Fluids.

Lungs

- Control dispersion of pure part of Body Fluids (coming from Spleen) to the space under the skin.
- Send part of fluids down to the Kidneys & Bladder.
- Said to "regulate the Water Passages".

Kidneys

Extremely important in physiology of Blood Fluids. Vaporize some of the fluids they receive and send back to Lungs to moisten Lungs.

Kidney Yang controls many stages of the transformation of fluids:

- Provides heat for Spleen to transform Body Fluids.
- Assists Small Intestine in its function to separate pure and impure Body Fluids.
- Provides Qi to Bladder for its function of Qi transformation.
- Assists Triple Burner (San Jiao) transformation and excretion of fluids.

Bladder

- Separates fluids it receives into pure and impure.
- Excretes urine with help of Kidney Yang.

San Jiao (Triple Burner)

Assists transformation, transportation and excretion of fluids at all stages.

- Upper Burner: is compared to a "mist": Lungs disperse fluids to the space under the skin.
- Middle Burner: is compared to a "muddy pool" (also to a "foam"). Stomach churns fluids and directs impure part to Small Intestine and pure part to Spleen.
- Lower Burner: compared to a "drainage ditch" or "swamp". Small Intestine separates pure from impure, Bladder and Kidneys transform, separate and excrete fluids.

Relationship between Qi and the Jin Ye

Qi transforms and transports fluids, otherwise fluids accumulate.

Qi holds the body fluids in, as it does with the blood. When the Qi is deficient, fluids can leak out.

Examples:

- Kidney Yang Deficiency causing Enuresis.
- Lung Qi Deficiency causing Spontaneous Sweating.
- Spleen Qi Deficiency causing Chronic Vaginal Discharge.

Qi is also dependant on Fluids, and a loss of FLuids can result in a deficiency of Qi.

Examples:

- Excessive sweating causes a loss of Defensive (Wei) Qi along with the Fluids.
- Excessive vomiting depletes Qi.

Relationship between Blood and the Jin Ye

Mutual nourishment:

- Body Fluids constantly replenish Blood and "thin it out" so that it does not coagulate. "If Body Fluids are harmonized they turn red and are transformed into Blood."
- Blood also nourishes Body Fluids: both are Yin. Hence loss of Fluids, e.g. in excessive perspiration, can cause Deficient Blood. Conversely, chronic blood loss can cause loss of Fluids and dryness.

Blood & Body Fluids have the same source and mutually nourish each other. In treatment, one should never cause sweating where a patient is bleeding or if there is significant Deficiency of Blood. Also one should never let blood when a patient is sweating.

ZANG-FU OR VISCERA

The Zang-fu is a collection organs that produce and regulate qi within the body. Unlike in western medicine, these organs should not be thought of as anatomical structures, but rather as interconnected functions that explain how qi is produced within the body. The functions performed by each organ are referred to as the organ's qi (i.e. Heart qi). In total, there are 11 organs, five Zang and six fu.

Zang refers to the five organs that are yin. Collectively, their primary purpose is to produce and store qi, xue (blood), Jinye (body fluids), Jing (essence), and shen (Spirit). They are the:

- Heart: Responsible for storing shen. Physically, it governs blood and the meridians. Emotionally, it controls joy.
- Spleen: The Spleen is one of the most dynamic organs. It is responsible for the transportation of essential qi and xue (blood) from nutrition and water, and actuating them to the other Zang It also helps to contain xue within the meridians. Physically, it governs the limbs. Emotionally, it controls pondering.
- Lung: The primary function of the lung is the actuation of pectoral qi, which is produced by breathing. Physically, it governs the skin and hair. Emotionally, it controls grief.
- Kidney: The kidney is a dynamic organ. It is responsible for the containment of shi, which guides conception, development, birth, and growth. Physically, it is responsible for producing marrow.
- Liver: The primary function of the liver is to ensure that qi can flow freely through the meridians. It also stores blood and maintains the tendons.

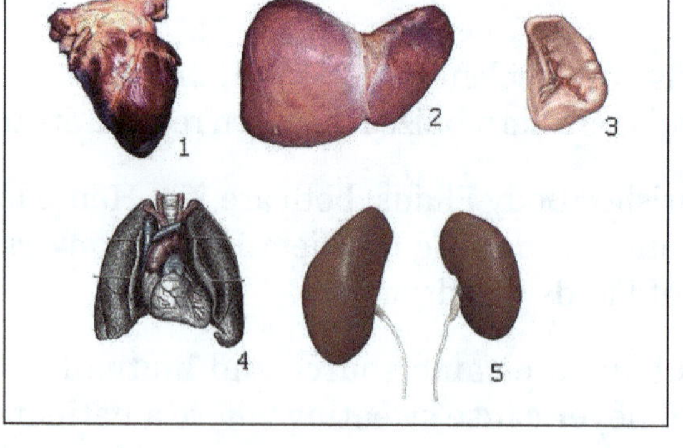

fu refers to six organs that are yang. Collectively, their primary function is to transmit and digest nutrients without storing them and to excrete waste. They are:

- Stomach: The stomach is considered to be of primary importance in TCM. It is here that food and water are first digested and nutritional qi is extracted. After food is digested, it is sent to the small intestine, for further purification.
- Small Intestine: The small intestine connects with the stomach and its main function is to further purify the nutrition that was partially digested by the stomach from a turbid into a clear substance. After purification, it transports the clear substance throughout the body, while expelling the turbid.
- Large Intestine: It's primary function is to receive waste material from the small intestine and to absorb any remaining good fluids while transforming the remaining waste into feces.
- Urinary Bladder: As the small intense purifies fluids, its sends turbid fluids to the urinary bladder, whose primary function is to store and discharge urine.
- Gall Bladder: The gall bladder is attached to the liver and its primary function is to transform any of the liver's remaining qi into bile.
- Sanjiao: It should be noted that the Sanjiao does not have a Western anatomical equivalent. Roughly, it can be thought of as 3 placeholders/cavities or jiao for the organs within the body's trunk. The 3 jiao are:
    - Upper Jiao: Holds the heart and lung.
    - Middle Jiao: Holds the spleen and stomach.
    - Lower jiao: Holds the kidney and urinary bladder.

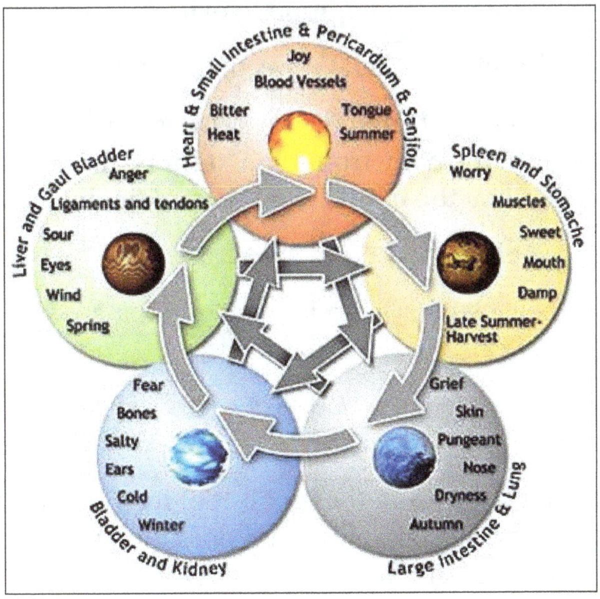

As mentioned earlier, each of the Zang-fu organs has a yin-yang pair and follows a Wu Xing cycle. Wu Xing, which translates into the Five Phases or Five Elements, is the notion that the change of the cosmos occurs in a cyclical pattern of five stages.

This means that each Zang-fu pair corresponds to one of the Five Elements and that they interact in a cyclical function with each other. The chart below helps demonstrate this relationship.

Table: The Five Fundamental Substances are what make and sustain life.

Element	Zang Organ(yin)	Fu Organ (yang)
Fire	Heart	Small Intestine
Earth	Spleen	Stomach
Metal	Lung	Large Intestine
Water	Kidney	Bladder
Wood	Liver	Gall Bladder

JING-LUO OR CHANNELS OF COMMUNICATION

- Jing Luo are the main channels of communication and energy distribution in the body.
- Link interior Zang Fu organs with various tissues of superficial areas of the body.

In this way, they allow for internal adaptation to external change.

- They connect different superficial areas of the body.
- The Jing Luo are more external (more Yang) than the Zang Fu Organs. When pathogens penetrate the body from the Exterior, they usually penetrate the superficial channels, then the main channels, and finally the Zang Fu Organs.
- Jing Luo cover the entire body

Every part of the musculoskeletal system is related to a main meridian and its associated sub-meridians.

Via the main channel, every part of the body associated with a given internal Organ can be affected by imbalance in that Organ.

i.e. - The Bladder channel: connects the small toe, lateral aspect of foot and ankle, posterior aspect of leg, buttocks, sacroiliac and dorsal region, occiput, vertex, central frontal region and inner canthus of eye.

Knowing the pathway of the channels, we can make connections in symptoms as diverse as itchy eyes, occipital headaches, lumbar pain and spasms in the gastrocnemius. i.e. - the Heart channel begins in the axilla and ends on the small finger. It has long been noted in western biomedicine that in the case of myocardial infarction, the pain often travels along this channel. TCM provides a link between this external muscular pain and an imbalance in the associated internal Organ.

Distribution of the Jing Luo

Most superficial	Cutaneous Regions	
Deeper	Tendinomuscular Meridians in the musculature	Province of Wei energy - 1st line of defense and adaptation
Deeper	Luo Meridians	Associated with Main channels but are more superficial. Link Yin and Yang coupled pairs. Link Primary Meridians with surrounding tissues.
Deeper	Divergent Meridians	Reinforce the circulatory network of 12 Primary Meridians. Provide more functional contacts between Yin and Yang channels.
Deeper	12 Primary Meridians	Connect with Zang Fu Organs. Carry mainly Ying (Nutritive Qi) and Blood.
	8 Extra Vessels	CV GV and Chong Mai originate in Kidney Organ. The others connect with Principal channels.
		Function: strengthen association between channels and control, store and regulate Qi and blood of channels (reservoirs). Carry mainly Yuan Qi.

The sub-meridian system (superficial channels) has the main functions of maintaining normal function providing for adaptation to changes in the external environment. This adaptation can often occur without the circulation of Qi in the main Meridians being too affected.

There is much disagreement regarding the pathways of the Luo and Tendinomuscular channels. In any case, these channels do not have their own points but share points of the Primary Meridians. The flow of Qi through these channels is affected by needling points on the Principal channels.

MERIDIAN SYSTEM

The meridian system is a concept in traditional Chinese medicine (TCM) about a path through which the life-energy known as "qi" flows.

Despite ongoing research into the existence of meridians, no convincing scientific evidence has been put forward for their existence. Major proponents of their existence have also not come to any consensus as to how they might work or be tested in a scientific context.

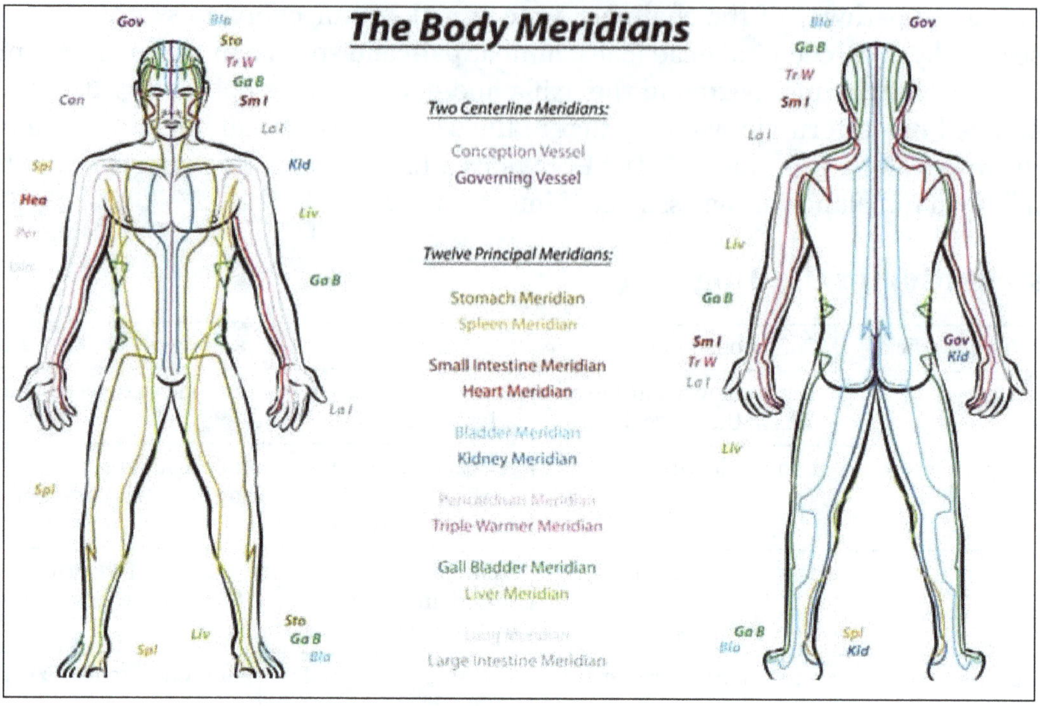

Meridian system.

The meridian network is typically divided into two categories, the jingmai or meridian channels and the luomai or associated vessels (sometimes called "collaterals"). The jingmai contain the 12 tendinomuscular meridians, the 12 divergent meridians, the 12 principal meridians, the eight extraordinary vessels as well as the Huato channel, a set of bilateral points on the lower back whose discovery is attributed to the ancient physician Hua Tuo. The collaterals contain 15 major arteries that connect the 12 principal meridians in various ways, in addition to the interaction with their associated internal organs and other related internal structures. The collateral system also incorporates a branching expanse of capillary-like vessels which spread throughout the body, namely in the 12 cutaneous regions as well as emanating from each point on the principal meridians. If one counts the number of unique points on each meridian, the total comes to 361, which matches the number of days in a year, in the moon calendar system. Note that this method ignores the fact that the bulk of acupoints are bilateral, making the actual total 670.

There are about 400 acupuncture points (not counting bilateral points twice) most of which are situated along the major 20 pathways (i.e. 12 primary and eight extraordinary channels). However, by the second Century AD, 649 acupuncture points were recognized in China (reckoned by counting bilateral points twice). There are "12 Principal Meridians" where each meridian corresponds to either a hollow or solid organ; interacting with it and extending along a particular extremity (i.e. arm or leg). There are also "Eight Extraordinary Channels", two of which have their own sets of points, and the remaining ones connecting points on other channels.

12 Standard Meridians

The 12 standard meridians, also called Principal Meridians, are divided into Yin and Yang groups. The Yin meridians of the arm are Lung, Heart, and Pericardium. The Yang meridians of the arm are Large Intestine, Small Intestine, and Triple Burner. The Yin Meridians of the leg are Spleen, Kidney, and Liver. The Yang meridians of the leg are Stomach, Bladder, and Gall Bladder.

Eight Extraordinary Meridians

The eight extraordinary meridians are of pivotal importance in the study of Qigong, T'ai chi ch'uan and Chinese alchemy. These eight extra meridians are different to the standard twelve organ meridians in that they are considered to be storage vessels or reservoirs of energy and are not associated directly with the Zang Fu, i.e. internal organs.

The eight extraordinary vessels are (qí jīng bā mài):

- Conception Vessel (Ren Mai).
- Governing Vessel (Du Mai).
- Penetrating Vessel (Chong Mai).
- Girdle Vessel (Dai Mai).
- Yin linking vessel (Yin Wei Mai).
- Yang linking vessel (Yang Wei Mai).
- Yin Heel Vessel (Yin Qiao Mai).
- Yang Heel Vessel (Yang Qiao Mai).

References

- Qi, principles, eng: shen-nong.com, Retrieved 6 January, 2020
- Xue-blood, wiki: tcmwiki.com, Retrieved 5 August, 2020
- What-is-zang-fu: amcollege.edu, Retrieved 2 July, 2020
- Acupuncture-channel-theory, get, acupuncture go: sacredlotus.com, Retrieved 1 April, 2020
- Novella, steven (25 january 2012). "what is traditional chinese medicine?". Sciencebasedmedicine.org. Society for science-based medicine. Retrieved 13 may 2015
- Jin-ye-body-fluids-vital-substance, get, foundations-chinese-medicine, go: sacredlotus.com, Retrieved 30 March, 2020
- Peter deadman and mazin al-khafaji with kevin baker. "a manuel of acupuncture" journal of chinese medicine, 2007. Isbn 978-0-9510546-5-9

The Theory of Yin and Yang

CHAPTER 3

Yin and Yang is a theory that describes how the opposite forces are interconnected, complementary and interdependent in the natural world. It divides the body organs into Yin and Yang. Yin organs include liver, heart, spleen, lung and kidney, while Yang organs are gall bladder, small intestine, stomach, large intestine, triple burner and urinary bladder. This chapter has been carefully written to provide an easy understanding of the theory of Yin and Yang.

Yin Yang is the concept of duality forming a whole. We encounter examples of Yin and Yang every day. As examples: night (Yin) and day (Yang), female (Yin) and male (Yang). Over thousands of years, quite a bit has been sorted and grouped under various Yin Yang classification systems.

The symbol for Yin Yang is called the Taijitu. Most people just call it the yin yang symbol in the west. The taijitu symbol has been found in more than one culture and over the years has come to represent Taoism.

Basic Concepts Defining the Nature of Yin Yang

- Neither Yin nor Yang is absolute: Nothing is completely Yin or completely Yang. Each aspect contains the beginning point for the other aspect. For example, day becomes night and then night becomes day. Yin and Yang are interdependent upon each other so that the definition of one requires the definition for the other to be complete.

- Yin Yang is not static: The nature of Yin and Yang flows and changes with time. A simple example is thinking about how the day gradually flows into the night. However, the length of day and night are changing. As the earth ages, its spin is slowing causing the length of day and night to get longer. Day and night are not static entities. Sometimes changes in the relationship between Yin and Yang can be dramatic where one aspect can just transform into the other. As an example: some species of fish have females that transform quickly into males when the population of males isn't enough.

- The summation of Yin and Yang form a whole. One effect of this is: as one aspect increases the other decreases to maintain the overall balance of the whole.

- The balance of Yin Yang can be skewed due to outside influences. Four possible imbalances exist:
    - Deficiency Yang.
    - Deficiency Yin.
    - Excess Yang.
    - Excess Yin.

These imbalances can be paired: so an excess of Yin can also simulate a Yang deficiency and vice versa.

As an example, this concept is especially important for Chinese healing practices. So an excess of Yang results in a fever. An excess of Yin could mean the accumulation of fluids in the body. Chinese healing examines a person's health by using the eight principles: Internal and External stimuli, Deficiency and Excesses, Cold and Heat and Yin and Yang.

- Yin Yang can be subdivided into additional Yin and Yang aspects. For example, a Yang aspect of Heat: can be further subdivided into a Yin warm or Yang burning.
- Additional principles that define Yin and Yang qualities exist. The concepts listed here are merely a starting point to illustrate the nature of Yin and Yang. Usually, as a practice, Taoism does a good job of not codifying life. Ironically, this wasn't true about yin Yang, since over history many Taoist's have tried to codify what is Yin and what is Yang. Typically Taoist texts will list a few examples of Yin and Yang and then meander off to the next topic. As an example go back to the Taoist passage quoted above from the Tao Te Ching. You will discover a few additional aspects to Yin and Yang, but the reading isn't a complete definition either. The author of this passage fully expects you as the reader to go out and to explore the ideas on your own.
- You can infinitely dig into Yin Yang due to its relative nature.

How Yin Yang Flows

Now forget everything you have learned about Yin and Yang for a moment. Step back from all the descriptions and classifications of Yin and Yang to consider the following passage from the Tao Te Ching:

- The Way begot one.
- And the one, two.
- Then the two begot three.
- And three, all else.

A clearer understanding of Yin Yang requires looking back into the Tao. The Tao can be considered as the fundamental absolute. Upon examination: the nature of the Tao expands out. This process of expansion defines a pattern, splitting apart into finer and finer patterns. Yin and Yang is the point where perception demarks the Tao's expansion into one and then one into two.

Taoism as a practice enjoys examining patterns. Over the years countless sects of Taoism have formed and quite a bit of literature written over the delineation and description of these patterns. Often Taoists use the concept of Yin Yang as a familiar starting template to work with patterns.

For example, Qigong is based on the patterns of breath and physical movement. Knowledge of bodily patterns forms the basis of this Taoist practice to keep a body healthy. The human body and its movements are divided according to Yin and Yang categories. So the upper body corresponds to the Yang, while the lower body roots into the Yin. The body's center is where the Yin and Yang meet. Qi Gong exercises are grouped and explained in terms of Yin and Yang to help classify the body's harmonies into a working practice. Knowledge of Yin or Yang isn't required to perform Qi Gong. Instead, it's an additional filter which helps people connect to the practice.

Another example is Taoist divination within the Book of Changes / I Ching. Divination in Taoism is a practice of examining human interactions based on well known psychological patterns. To generate a result either coins or yarrow stalks are tossed down to form a pattern. The patterns generated correspond to Yin and Yang defined qualities. The nature of the Yin and Yang pattern is applied to the psychology of the moment to return advice for the person asking the question.

Yin Yang is a fundamental aspect of Taoist thought. We always naturally apply human-based values over naturally occurring patterns. However, remember it's also important not to chase finer and finer descriptions of these patterns, to do so would be to chase down infinity.

Yin Yang is a system of recognizing how to separate out patterns in our life while also relaxing to accept the overall whole and complete nature of the Tao.

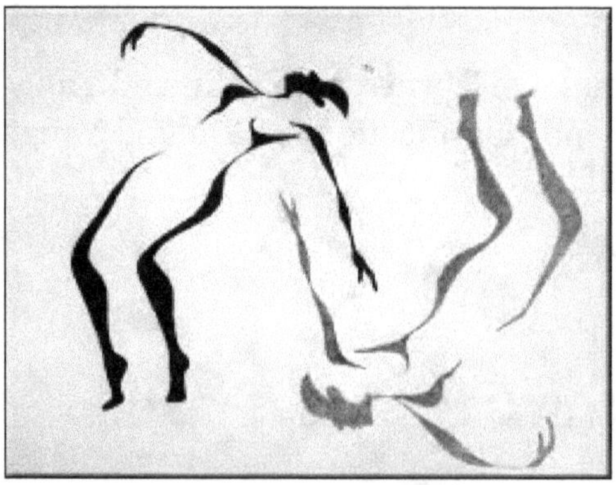

Yin and Yang of Spirit and Soul.

The Yin and Yang nature of soul and spirit. We travel between these two poles of our nature.

It's a trap to think of life as only being a single aspect of ourselves: when in actuality we spin in the yin and yang nature of many aspects.

To grab on tightly to only one part of one's nature creates a dam: upon which rides a flood of chaos: as the larger momentum of the universe will then always pick up to kick things about.

YIN ORGANS

Liver

In western physiology, the liver is responsible for a number of important body functions, including the production and excretion of bile, which is used to break down fat and the detoxification of blood. However, according to TCM, the liver's functions are different. They include control of the central nervous system, the autonomic nervous system (the part of the nervous system over which a person does not have voluntary control), and the circulatory system. In addition, the liver is responsible for vision.

"The liver rules flowing and spreading."

In TCM, the liver promotes flowing and spreading movements. By stimulating flow, the liver adjusts and ensures the smooth movement of qi, blood and body fluids, and spreads these substances to the entire body. There are three functional aspects of the liver's "flowing and spreading" activity: regulating qi, regulating emotions and enhancing the digestive properties of the spleen.

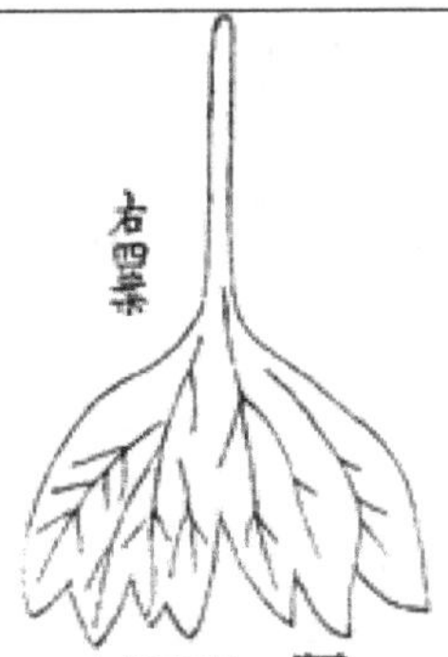

LIVER 肝

Regulating Qi Movement

The activities of the organs and meridians are dependent on qi movement. The flow and spread of qi throughout the body are in turn dependent on the regulatory functions of the liver. If the liver is not functioning properly, qi flow is interrupted, which can lead to disharmony and imbalance. When this becomes marked, disease and other health problems ensue.

Regulating Emotions

The liver balances emotions. Normal emotional health depends on the harmony of qi and blood. When the liver keeps qi flowing smoothly, a relaxed internal, emotional environment is created. If liver disharmony results in stagnant liver qi, emotional disturbances like depression and anger can occur.

Enhancing the Digestive Power of Spleen

The liver's flowing and spreading functions also adjust the digestive functions of spleen. If the liver is not functioning properly, the movement of spleen qi is not smooth. Consequently, the transformation and transportation of digested food will be affected, leading to abdominal pain, nausea, belching, diarrhea and other complications.

"The liver stores the blood."

The liver is also responsible for storing and regulating blood flow. When a person moves or exercises, the blood leaves the liver and goes to the part of body that needs it. The blood returns to the liver to be stored, when a person rests. If a person has insufficient blood available for storage in the liver, their eyes will not be adequately nourished and will become rough and dry. Dizziness can also occur.

"The liver opens into the eyes."

The eyes have a close relationship with the liver; because, they are connected to the liver meridian. The ability to see depends on the nourishment of the eyes from blood stored in the liver, and many liver disorders are reflected in the eyes. For example, insufficient liver blood can lead to blurred vision. "Dampness and heat" of the liver and gall bladder, a condition known in western medicine as jaundice, manifests as yellow eyes.

"The liver rules the tendons and is manifested in the nails."

The proper movement of tendons, which attach muscle to bone, is closely related to liver function. If the blood stored in the liver is insufficient and incapable of nourishing the tendons, symptoms like spasms, numbness of limbs and difficulty bending or stretching occur. Fingernail and toenail health is also dependent on the nourishment of blood from the liver. If the liver blood is sufficient, nails will appear pink and moist. If it is insufficient, the nails will become thin, brittle and pale.

Heart

In TCM, the functions of the heart are different from those of the anatomical heart, as it is understood in western medicine. The heart organ represents a group of physiological functions. In addition to regulating the cardiovascular system, it is responsible for maintaining the nervous system's functions.

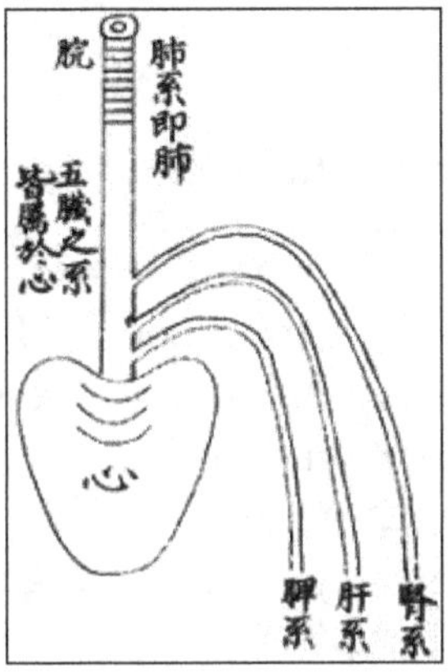

"The heart rules the blood and blood vessels".

The heart is the functional unit for regulating blood flow. Blood is transported inside the blood vessels around the entire body when the heart pumps. The heart, blood and blood vessels are united by their common activities. In TCM, this functional relationship is known as the "ruling" of the heart.

Heart qi refers to the pumping actions of the heart. If heart qi is abundant and sufficient, the heart pumps at a normal pace, transporting blood smoothly inside the blood vessels, the pulse is regular and strong, and the face will look brilliant. As a result, the body is able to obtain from blood the nutrients needed to sustain life. On the other hand, if heart qi is deficient, blood cannot maintain an efficient flow in the blood vessels, and the pulse is weak. The individual looks pale, and the tongue also appears pale and white. Without healthy ruling of the heart, individuals will experience palpitations, chest discomfort and pain.

"The heart rules the spirit"

In TCM, the heart stores the "spirit". In general, the "spirit" refers to an individual's vitality, which is reflected in the eyes, speech, reactions and overall appearance. Specifically, the "spirit" refers to a person's mental, cognitive and intellectual abilities. The heart takes charge of mental activities by mastering other organs and their physiological functions. If the "spirit ruling" is good, the individual will be wise and have a clear and fast mind. If there is heart disharmony, signs like forgetfulness, poor self esteem, and slow thought processes or reactions occur.

"Sweat is the fluid of the heart."

Sweat comes from body fluids, which are an essential and integral part of blood. Blood is ruled by the heart and is the main fluid of this organ. Because sweat comes from the same origin as blood, in TCM over-sweating is considered an exploitation of qi and heart blood, leading to symptoms such as palpitations. As a result, people who sweat abnormally usually have a heart deficiency. If such sweating is spontaneous, the disharmony belongs to a deficiency of heart yang. If it takes place at night, the disharmony belongs to a deficiency of heart yin.

“The heart opens into the tongue. The heart’s brilliance is manifested in the face.”

In TCM, both the tongue and face are windows for the heart and blood. The heart “opens into the tongue” because they are connected. By observing the tongue and looking for the “heart’s brilliance to be manifested in the face, ” a lot can be learned about how the heart is functioning. For example, if heart function is normal, individuals will have bright, healthy red cheeks and the tongue will appear pink. If there is blood stasis (where blood is not able to flow smoothly through the blood vessels), the face and tongue will appear purple. A healthy blood supply is also essential for providing nutrients for hair growth, because in TCM, hair is thought to be the “remains of blood.” If hair growth is affected, it may indicate a problem with the heart and blood.

Spleen

In western physiology, the spleen is a large, vascular, lymphatic organ. It acts as a reservoir and filters the blood. It also plays a role in making blood early on in life. In TCM, the spleen does not perform these functions. It assists with digestion, blood coagulation and fluid metabolism in the body.

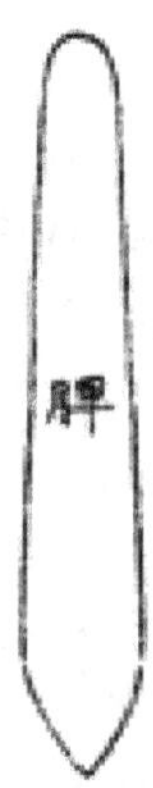

SPLEEN 脾

“The spleen rules transformation and transportation.”

Since the spleen is the primary organ responsible for digestion, its main function is to transform food into essence used for qi and blood transformation. Once the ingested food and liquids get into the body, the spleen extracts a pure nutritive essence from them. This pure nutritive essence is used for the production of qi, blood and body fluids, which the spleen then transports throughout the body. Liquids extracted as pure nutritive essence are sent upwards to the lung for dissemination and redistribution. However, some will descend to the kidney and bladder to be excreted as urine.

If the transformation and transportation functions of the spleen are harmonious, there will be abundant nutritive essence for qi and blood, but if the spleen is in disharmony, its digestive powers will be affected. As a result, abdominal distention, pain, diarrhea or malaise occurs.

"The spleen rules ascending pure essence."

After transforming food into nutritive essence, the spleen sends it upwards to the heart and lungs where it is transformed into qi and blood for nourishment of the whole body. Food not transformed into nutritive essence becomes an impure substance. While the spleen ascends pure essence, the stomach, (the spleen's corresponding exterior organ), will descend the impure substances inside the digestive tract. By ascending the pure nutritive essence and descending the impure substances, a balance in the digestive system is created.

"The spleen governs the blood."

Not only does the spleen transform food essence, it also governs the movement of blood by keeping it flowing in its proper pathways in the blood vessels. When spleen qi is sufficient, there is adequate production of qi and blood, and blood is, therefore, kept inside the blood vessels. If the spleen's functions are in disharmony, the blood escapes from its normal pathways, leading to symptoms such as bloody vomit, blood in the stool, blood under the skin, blood in urine, or menorrhagia (excessive menstrual bleeding).

"The spleen rules the muscles and flesh. It opens into the mouth and its brilliance is manifested in the lips."

In TCM, the movements of the muscles and the four limbs depend on the power of the spleen. When spleen qi is sufficient, the limbs and muscles are healthy and strong because they are nourished by the blood and qi. If spleen qi is deficient, however, the muscles become weak and an individual may feel tired and have general malaise.

The lips and mouth are also affected by the spleen's health. If spleen function is harmonious, the mouth can distinguish the five tastes (sweet, salty, sour, bitter and pungent (spicy)), and the lips appear red and moist. If the spleen is weak, the mouth cannot distinguish the different tastes and the lips will be pale.

Lungs

In western physiology, the lungs are responsible for air exchange. In addition to performing respiration in TCM, the lungs' regulate fluid metabolism, blood circulation, the autonomic nervous system and the immune system.

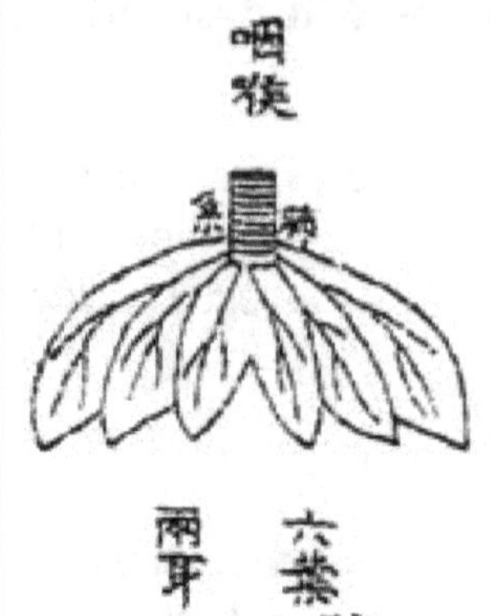

LUNGS 肺

"The lungs rule qi and administer respiration."

The lungs are where qi exchange and regulation occurs. During inhalation, the lungs take in natural air qi (one type of qi referring to the atmospheric air), propelling it downward where it meets other types of qi. The different types of qi combine to produce normal qi (qi present in the body). During exhalation, the lung expels the "impure" air not useful to the body. If the lungs are healthy, qi will enter the body smoothly and respiration will be even and regular. If there is lung disharmony, respiration is weakened and normal qi production is affected, leading to qi deficiency.

"The lungs direct movement in a disseminating, descending and liquefying manner."

The lungs disseminate substances in an ascending and outward direction. For example, impure air is expelled in this manner, and body fluids and food nutritive essence are directed towards the skin and hair. By regulating sweat secretion, the lungs disseminate protective qi (qi mainly responsible for immunity) to the skin and the pores.

The lungs also demonstrate descending and liquefying properties. They take in natural air qi during respiration and liquefy the fluids in the airway. The lungs then descend these substances downwards along with food essence transformed by the spleen. The descending function is necessary to maintain a normal respiratory tract.

The disseminating, descending and liquefying properties of the lungs are essential for good health. If disharmony occurs, individuals may suffer from coughing, wheezing, chest discomfort, abnormal sweating or congestion from phlegm.

"The lungs move and adjust the water channels".

The lungs are responsible for the transformation and movement of water in the body. They move water in the same directions as qi. The lungs' disseminating properties enable water vapor to ascend and scatter to the skin pores. This is the process of normal sweating. The lungs also liquefy and cause water vapor to descend to the kidneys, where the liquefied waste is excreted as urine.

Large Intestine

The large intestine receives the "impure" parts of the digested food from the small intestine and continues to absorb water from these materials. At the end of the process, stools are formed and excreted through the anus. Large intestine disharmony presents with symptoms of abdominal pain, intestinal rumblings and diarrhea. Sometimes, if there is excessive "heat", intestinal fluids will dry up, and constipation will occur.

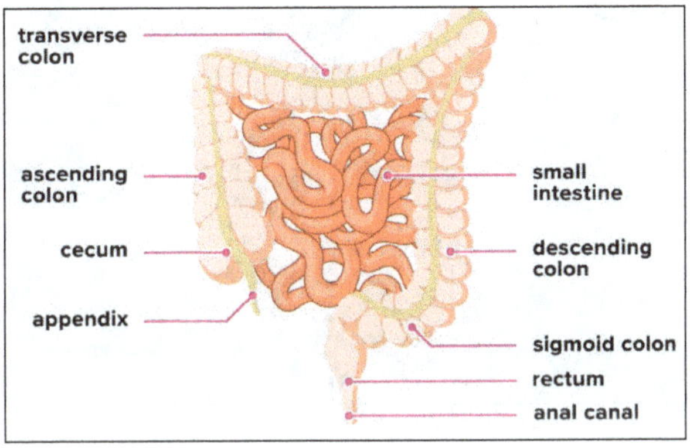

Bladder

The bladder is responsible for storing and excreting urine. As previously discussed, the lungs, spleen and kidneys all have roles in fluid metabolism and regulating the water distribution in the body. The "turbid' water collected by the kidneys that cannot be reused by the body is sent to the bladder for excretion as urine. TCM describes this function as "vaporization" of urine in the bladder. Disharmony of the bladder can lead to urinary problems such as incontinence or difficult urination. Kidney function complements bladder function so a problem with the bladder often indicates kidney problems as well.

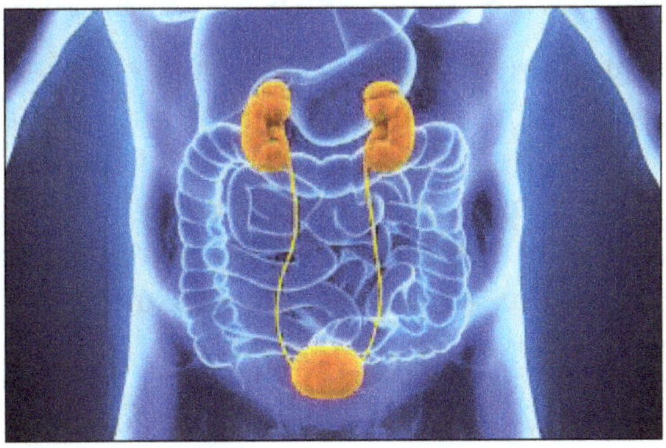

Triple Burner

The triple burner is a special concept in TCM, and there is no corresponding organ in western medicine. Suggestions have been made that the triple burner's function may be related to the pancreas and metabolism in the body, but no clear conclusion has been reached as to the nature of this organ. The triple burner is actually a collective term for the upper, middle and lower burner. The Chinese word "triple burner" actually means "three parts which burn or scorch."

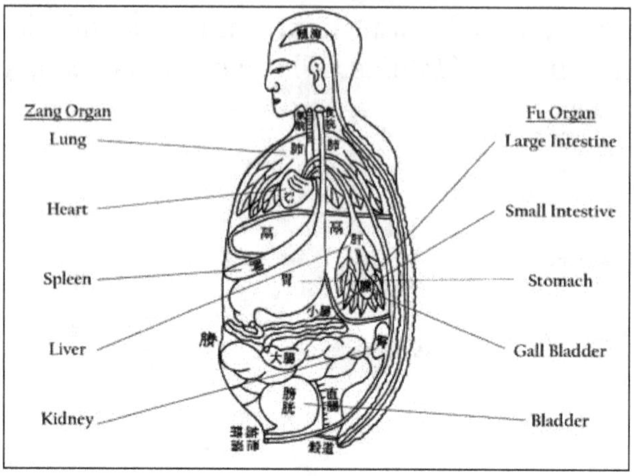

The upper burner is located above the diaphragm and includes the heart and lungs. The middle burner is located in the region above the belly button and below the diaphragm and includes the spleen and stomach. The lower burner is located below the belly button, and it includes the liver, kidneys, large intestine, small intestine and bladder. (This description of location is used for the functional classification of the TCM triple burner. The above locations do not refer to the anatomical location of organs.)

The triple burner's functions relate to the activities of qi and the movement of water. The functions of the three burners were summarized in the Huang Di Nei Jing (The Yellow Emperor's Classic of Internal Medicine) as follows: "The upper burner acts like a mist. The middle burner acts like foam. The lower burner acts like a swamp."

"Mist" refers to the disseminating functions of the upper burner. With this function, qi, blood and body fluids are distributed throughout the body just as mist disperses in the environment. "Foam" means the digestive churning of the middle burner. When the spleen and stomach transform and ripen food, the food decomposes in a similar way to foaming. "Swamp" relates to the excretion of impure substances. The lower burner separates the "clear" from the "turbid" substances and excretes these impurities as wastes- like a swamp breaks down certain vegetation.

The triple burner is the passage through which water, food and fluid are transported. The Huang Di Nei Jing (The Yellow Emperor's Classic of Internal Medicine) also says, "The triple burner is the controller of the entire circulation of body fluid". Therefore, disharmony of the triple burner can lead to edema (fluid collection in the tissues) or difficult urination. Treatment of these conditions is aimed at resuming the harmony of the affected organs such as the lungs, spleen or kidneys.

Linguistic Aspects

These Chinese terms yin "shady side" and yang "sunny side" are linguistically analyzable in terms of Chinese characters, pronunciations and etymology, meanings, topography, and loanwords.

Characters

The Traditional Chinese characters and for the words yīn and yáng are both classified as radical-phonetic characters, combining the semantically significant "mound; hill" radical or with the phonetic indicators ying and yang. The first phonetic yīn "cloudy" ideographically combines jīn "now; present" and yún "cloud", denoting the " presence of clouds". The second phonetic yáng "bright" originally pictured the "sun" with "rays coming down". This phonetic is expanded with the "sun" radical into yáng "rising sun; sunshine". The "mound; hill" radical full forms semantically specify yīn "shady/dark side of a hill" and yáng "sunny/light side of a hill".

The Simplified Chinese characters and for yīn and yáng combine the same "hill" radical with the non-phonetic yuè "moon" and rì "sun", graphically denoting "shady side of a hill" and "sunny side of a hill". Compare the Classical Chinese names (which contain tài "great") for these two heavenly bodies: Tàiyīn "moon" and Tàiyáng "sun".

Pronunciations and Etymologies

The Modern Standard Chinese pronunciation of or is usually level first tone yīn "shady; cloudy" or sometimes falling fourth tone yìn "to shelter; shade", and or "sunny" is always pronounced with rising second tone yáng.

Sinologists and historical linguists have reconstructed Middle Chinese pronunciations from data in the Qieyun rhyme dictionary and later rhyme tables, which was subsequently used to reconstruct Old Chinese phonology from rhymes in the Shijing and phonological components of Chinese characters. Reconstructions of Old Chinese have illuminated the etymology of modern Chinese words.

Compare these Middle Chinese and Old Chinese (with asterisk) reconstructions of yīn and yáng:

- ·iəm < *·iəm and iang < *diang (Bernhard Karlgren).
- *ʔjəm and *raŋ (Li Fang-Kuei).
- ʔ(r)jum and *ljang (William H. Baxter).
- ʔjəm < *ʔəm and jiaŋ < *laŋ (Axel Schuessler).
- 'im < *qrum and yang < *laŋ (William H. Baxter and Laurent Sagart).

Schuessler gives probable Sino-Tibetan etymologies for both Chinese words.

Yin < *ʔəm compares with Burmese ʔum[C] "overcast; cloudy", Adi muk-jum "shade", and Lepcha so'yŭm "shade"; and is probably cognate with Chinese àn < *ʔə̂m? "dim; gloomy" and qīn < *khəm "blanket".

Yang < *laŋ compares with Lepcha a-lóŋ "reflecting light", Burmese laŋ[B] "be bright" and ə-laŋ[B] "light"; and is perhaps cognate with Chinese chāng < *k-hlaŋ "prosperous; bright" (compare areal words like Tai plaŋ[A1] "bright" & Proto-Viet-Muong hlaŋ[B]). To this word-family, Unger also includes bĭng < *pl(j)aŋ? "bright"; however Schuessler reconstructs Old Chinese pronunciation as *braŋ? and includes it in an Austroasiatic word family, besides liàng < *raŋh shuăng < *sraŋ? "twilight (of dawn)"; míng < mraŋ "bright, become light, enlighten"; owing to "the different OC initial consonant which seems to have no recognizable OC morphological function".

Meanings

Yin and yang are semantically complex words.

John DeFrancis's Chinese-English dictionary gives the following translation equivalents.

Yin or Noun ① [philosophy] negative/passive/female principle in nature ② Surname Bound morpheme ① the moon ② shaded orientation ③ covert; concealed; hidden ④ ⑦ negative ⑧ north side of a hill ⑨ south bank of a river ⑩ reverse side of a stele ⑪in intaglio Stative verb ① overcast

Yang Bound morpheme ① [Chinese philosophy] positive/active/male principle in nature ②the sun ④ in relief ⑤ open; overt ⑥ belonging to this world ⑦ [linguistics] masculine ⑧ south side of a hill ⑨ north bank of a river

The compound yinyang or means "yin and yang; opposites; ancient Chinese astronomy; occult arts; astrologer; geomancer; etc.".

The sinologist Rolf Stein etymologically translates Chinese yin "shady side (of a mountain)" and yang "sunny side (of a mountain)" with the uncommon English geographic terms ubac "shady side of a mountain" and adret "sunny side of a mountain" (which are of French origin).

Toponymy

Many Chinese place names or toponyms contain the word yang "sunny side" and a few contain yin "shady side". In China, as elsewhere in the Northern Hemisphere, sunlight comes predominantly from the south, and thus the south face of a mountain or the north bank of a river will receive more direct sunlight than the opposite side.

Yang refers to the "south side of a hill" in Hengyang, which is south of Mount Heng in Hunan province, and to the "north bank of a river" in Luoyang, which is located north of the Luo River in Henan.

Similarly, yin refers to "north side of a hill" in Huayin, which is north of Mount Hua in Shaanxi province.

In Japan, the characters are used in western Honshu to delineate the north-side San'in region from the south-side San'yō region, separated by the Chūgoku Mountains.

Loanwords

English yin, yang, and yin-yang are familiar loanwords of Chinese origin.

yin (jɪn) Also Yin, Yn. [Chinese yīn shade, feminine; the moon.]

a. In Chinese philosophy, the feminine or negative principle (characterized by dark, wetness, cold, passivity, disintegration, etc.) of the two opposing cosmic forces into which creative energy divides and whose fusion in physical matter brings the phenomenal world into being. Also attrib. or as adj., and transf. Cf. yang.

b. Comb., as yin-yang, the combination or fusion of the two cosmic forces; freq. attrib., esp. as yin-yang symbol, a circle divided by an S-shaped line into a dark and a light segment, representing respectively yin and yang, each containing a 'seed' of the other.

yang (jæŋ) Also Yang. [Chinese yáng yang, sun, positive, male genitals.]

a. In Chinese philosophy, the masculine or positive principle (characterized by light, warmth, dryness, activity, etc.) of the two opposing cosmic forces into which creative energy divides and whose fusion in physical matter brings the phenomenal world into being. Also attrib. or as adj. Cf. yin.

b. Comb.: yang-yin = yin-yang s.v. yin b.

For the earliest recorded "yin and yang" usages, the OED cites 1671 for yin and yang, 1850 for yin-yang, and 1959 for yang-yin.

In English, yang-yin (like ying-yang) occasionally occurs as a mistake or typographical error for the Chinese loanword yin-yang— yet they are not equivalents. Chinese does have some yangyin collocations, such as (lit. "foreign silver") "silver coin/dollar", but not even the most comprehensive dictionaries (e.g., the Hanyu Da Cidian) enter yang-yin *. While yang and yin can occur together in context, yangyin is not synonymous with yinyang. The linguistic term "irreversible binomial" refers to a collocation of two words A-B that cannot be idiomatically reversed as B-A, for example, English cat and mouse (not *mouse and cat) and friend or foe (not *foe or friend).

Similarly, the usual pattern among Chinese binomial compounds is for positive A and negative B, where the A word is dominant or privileged over B, for example, tiandi "heaven and earth" and nannü "men and women". Yinyang meaning "dark and light; female and male; moon and sun", however, is an exception. Scholars have proposed various explanations for why yinyang violates this pattern, including "linguistic convenience" (it is easier to say yinyang than yangyin), the idea that "proto-Chinese society was matriarchal", or perhaps, since yinyang first became prominent during the late Warring States period, this term was "purposely directed at challenging persistent cultural assumptions".

Nature

In Daoist philosophy, dark and light, yin and yang, arrive in the Tao Te Ching. It becomes sensible from an initial quiescence or emptiness (wuji, sometimes symbolized by an empty circle), and continues moving until quiescence is reached again. For instance, dropping a stone in a calm pool of water will simultaneously raise waves and lower troughs between them, and this alternation of high and low points in the water will radiate outward until the movement dissipates and the pool is calm once more. Yin and yang thus are always opposite and equal qualities. Further, whenever one quality reaches its peak, it will naturally begin to transform into the opposite quality: for example, grain that reaches its full height in summer (fully yang) will produce seeds and die back in winter (fully yin) in an endless cycle.

It is impossible to talk about yin or yang without some reference to the opposite, since yin and yang are bound together as parts of a mutual whole (for example, there cannot be the bottom of the foot without the top). A way to illustrate this idea is to postulate the notion of a race with only men or only women; this race would disappear in a single generation. Yet, men and women together create new generations that allow the race they mutually create (and mutually come from) to survive. The interaction of the two gives birth to things, like manhood. Yin and yang transform each other: like an undertow in the ocean, every advance is complemented by a retreat, and every rise transforms into a fall. Thus, a seed will sprout from the earth and grow upwards towards the sky—an intrinsically yang movement. Then, when it reaches its full potential height, it will fall. Also, the growth of the top seeks light, while roots grow in darkness.

Certain catchphrases have been used to express yin and yang complementarity:

- The bigger the front, the bigger the back.
- Illness is the doorway to health.
- Tragedy turns to comedy.
- Disasters turn out to be blessings.

Symbolism and Importance

Yin is the black side with the white dot in it, and yang is the white side with the black dot in it. The relationship between yin and yang is often described in terms of sunlight playing over a mountain and a valley. Yin (literally the 'shady place' or 'north slope') is the dark area occluded by the mountain's bulk, while yang (literally the "sunny place' or "south slope") is the brightly lit portion. As the sun moves across the sky, yin and yang gradually trade places with each other, revealing what was obscured and obscuring what was revealed.

Yin is characterized as slow, soft, yielding, diffuse, cold, wet, and passive; and is associated with water, earth, the moon, femininity, and night time.

Yang, by contrast, is fast, hard, solid, focused, hot, dry, and active; and is associated with fire, sky, the sun, masculinity and daytime.

Yin and yang also applies to the human body. In traditional Chinese medicine good health is directly related to the balance between yin and yang qualities within oneself. If yin and yang become unbalanced, one of the qualities is considered deficient or has vacuity.

I Ching

In the I Ching, originally a divination manual of the Western Zhou period, yin and yang are represented by broken and solid lines: yin is broken (⚋) and yang is solid (⚊). These are then combined into trigrams, which are more yang (e.g. ☱) or more yin (e.g. ☳) depending on the number of broken and solid lines (e.g., ☰ is heavily yang, while ☷ is heavily yin), and trigrams are combined into hexagrams (e.g. ⚊ and ⚊). The relative positions and numbers of yin and yang lines within the trigrams determines the meaning of a trigram, and in hexagrams the upper trigram is considered yang with respect to the lower trigram, yin, which allows for complex depictions of interrelations.

Taijitu

The principle of yin and yang is represented by the Taijitu (literally "Diagram of the Supreme Ultimate"). The term is commonly used to mean the simple "divided circle" form, but may refer to any of several schematic diagrams representing these principles, such as the swastika, common to Hinduism, Buddhism, and Jainism. Similar symbols have also appeared in other cultures, such as in Celtic art and Roman shield markings.

Taijiquan

Taijiquan, a form of martial art, is often described as the principles of yin and yang applied to the human body and an animal body. Wu Jianquan, a famous Chinese martial arts teacher, described Taijiquan as follows:

> Various people have offered different explanations for the name Taijiquan. Some have said: – 'In terms of self-cultivation, one must train from a state of movement towards a state of stillness. Taiji comes about through the balance of yin and yang. In terms of the art of attack and defense then, in the context of the changes of full and empty, one is constantly internally latent, to not outwardly expressive, as if the yin and yang of Taiji have not yet divided apart.' Others say: 'Every movement of Taijiquan is based on circles, just like the shape of a Taijitu. Therefore, it is called Taijiquan.
>
> —Wu Jianquan

THE OPPOSITION AND INTERDEPENDENCE OF YIN AND YANG

The opposition of yin and yang generalizes the contradiction and struggle of the two opposites within an object or phenomenon. Ancient scholars used water and fire to symbolize the basic properties of yin and yang. That is to say, the basic properties of yin simulate those water, including coldness, downward direction, dimness, etc., while the basic properties of yang are like those of fire, including hotness, upward direction, brightness, etc. From this, it can bi inferred that anything that has the characteristics of quiescence, coldness, lower position (or downward direction), interior position (or inward direction), dimness, asthenia, inhibition, slowness, or which is substantial, etc., pertains to ying whereas anything that is moving, hot, in an upper position (or moving in an upward direction), exterior position (or outward), bright, sthenic, excited, rapid, non-substantial etc., belongs to yang.

Since the yin-yang nature of a thing exists only bay comparison, and moreover that a thing can be divided infinitely, its yin-yang nature is by no means absolute, but its relative. In some circumstances the two opposites of a thing may change, and so the yin-yang nature of the thing also changes. There exist the conditions of a yin aspect developing within yin, yang within yang, yang complicated with yin, and yin complicated with yang. This concept conforms with objective reality.

The tissues and organs of the human body may pertain either to yin or yang according to their relative locations and functions. Viewing the body as a whole, the trunk surface and the four extremities, being on the exterior, pertain to yang, while the zang-fu organs are inside the body and are yin. Viewing the body surface and the four extremities alone, the back pertains to yang, while the chest and abdomen pertain to yin; the portion above the waist pertains to yang and that below pertains to yin; the lateral aspect of the four extremities pertains to yang and the medial aspect to yin; the channels running along the lateral aspect of an extremity pertain to yang, while those along the medial aspect pertain to yin. When speaking of the zang-fu organs alone, the fu organs with their main function of transmitting and digesting food pertain to yang; while the zang organs with their main function of storing vital essence and vital energy pertain to yin. Each of the zang-fu organs itself can again be divided into yin and yang, e.g., the yin and the yang of the kidney, the yin and the yang of the stomach, etc. In short, however complex the tissues and structures of the human body and their functional activities, the can be generalized and explained by the relation of yin and yang.

The interdependent relation of yin and yang means that each of the two aspects is the condition for the other's existence and neither of them can exist in isolation. For instance, without daytime there would be no night; without excitation there would be no inhibition. Hence, it can be seen that yin and yang are at once in opposition and in interdependence; they rely on each other for existence, coexisting in a single entity. The movement and change of a thing are due not only to the opposition and conflict between yin and yang but also to their relationship of interdependence and mutual support.

In physiological activities, the transformation of substance into function or vice versa verifies the theory of the interdepending relation of yin and yang. Substance pertains to yin and function to yang, the former being the basis of the latter, while the latter is the reflection of the existence of the former and also the motive force for the production of the former. Only when there are ample nutrient substances can the functional activities of the zang-fu organs are sound are they able constantly to stimulate the production of nutrient substances. The coordination and equilibrium between substance and function are the vital guarantee of physiological activities. Hence we find in Neijing: "Yin is installed in the interior as the material foundation of yang, while yang remains on the exterior as the manifestation of the function of yin."

References

- What-is-yin-yang, Taoism: personaltao.com, Retrieved 30 August, 2020
- Fiveyinorgans, principles, eng: shen-nong.com, Retrieved 13 April, 2020
- Feuchtwang, Stephan (2016). Religions in the Modern World: Traditions and Transformations. New York: Routledge. P. 150. ISBN 978-0-415-85881-6
- Sixyangorgans, principles eng: shen-nong.com, Retrieved 5 February, 2020
- The-opposition-and-interdependence-of-yin-and-yang: wordpress.com, Retrieved 3 May, 2020

The Five Elements

CHAPTER 4

Wu Xing are the five types of energies, dominating at different types. The names of the "Five Phases" are metal, wood, water, fire and earth. This chapter closely examines the elements of Wu Xing to provide an extensive understanding of the subject.

The Theory of the Five Eleme nts - Wu Xing , often shortened to Five Elements, is the concept in Chinese philosophy conceiving the world as dynamic states, or phases, of constant change.

Maybe the Taoistic theory of the Five Elements can be seen as a further, more refined step to understand and categorize or analyse the Yin-Yang philosophy.

The Theory of the Five Elements describes the interaction and relation between Yin and Yang, between phenomena.

Taoism theories use symbols to describe phenomens of reality, hence each of the Five Elements represent an aspect of a dynamic process, a processe's phases of change. In this sense, Wood is not only the actual wood of a tree as defined by the substance, but describes the character, the dynamic state, the elemental force of the element.

- Wood: Rising, development (of an action), impulse, expansion, decampment.
- Fire: Embodiement, definition, action, dynamic phase, design.
- Earth: Alteration, transformation, transmutation, change, convertation.
- Metal: Sinking, contraction, declining.
- Water: Contemplation, calmness, (re-)consideration, observation, reflection.

The basic substances of the material world according to the 'Theory of the Five Elements' are Wood, Fire, Earth, Metal and Water.

All material things are made of a single or a combination of the Five Elements, since these are the fundamental components.

All Five Elements are equally important and should form a balance, while being in constant move and cyclical change (phases).

Each phase's peak already consists of its decline, then forwarding the prior received/ gathered (chi) energy from one element to the following element.

The 'generating' or 'controlling' element is building up the energy to its own peak, before the decline starts again.

This interactive process is being constantly repeated, hence forming a never ending, though balanced circle.

Not only time changes things, but since everything changes within itself anyway, the 'Theory of the Five Element' is simply an observation of natural, creative changes; and it is the natural world confirming that all forces and energies in nature can be in constant smooth and harmonious transition from one phase to another - just as one season 'becomes' the next.

Each existing material, combined of parts of the Five Elements, shows a pre- domination of one of the Five Elements and is assigned an abstract generalization, hence can be classified accordingly.

Associations were later made with the human body and its organs and senses, colours, biota, foods etc. ("The East generates wind, wind generates wood, wood generates sour, sour generates liver, liver generates tendons".)

The Generating, Inter-Promoting or Enhancing Cycle (Shēng)

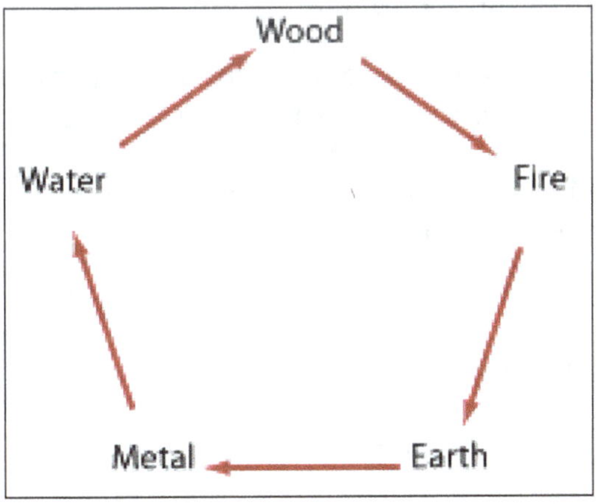

The Generating Cycle: one element (serving as parent) enriches, nourishes, strengthens, promotes growth and development of the following element (serving as child).

Generating: Wood feeds Fire - Fire creates Earth (ash) - Earth bears Metal - Metal (trace elements) collects, enrich Water - Water nourishes Wood.

Interpretation: (supporting, helping)

- Wood is the supporting element of Fire: Fire can release the power of Wood.

- Fire is the supporting element of Earth: Earth can release the power of Fire.
- Earth is the supporting element of Metal: Metal can release the power of Earth.
- Metal is the supporting element of Water: Water can release the power of Metal.
- Water is the supporting element of Wood: Wood can release the power of Water.

Controlling, Destructing/Inter-restraining and the Weakening Cycle

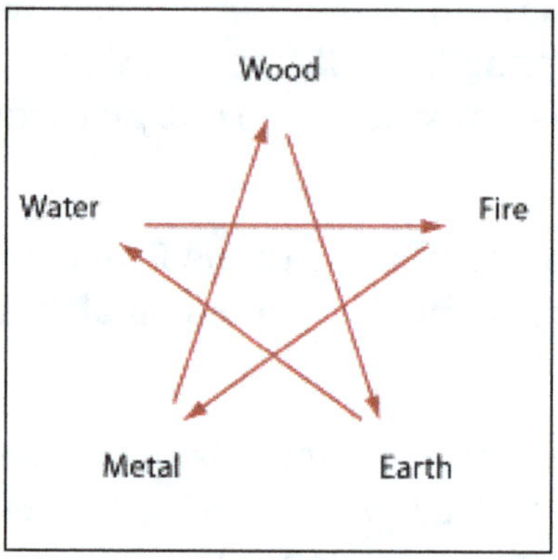

The Controling (Destructing) cycle.

Grandparent - Grandchild relationship: the controlling cycle provides for a check and balance system among all of the elements.

The controlling or destructing cycle: one element surpresses, controls, dominates, overcomes, weakens another element, preventing it from establishing its power.

A metalic knife can cut wood into pieces, hence controlling the shape of wood (though not destroying the chi energy).

Interpretation:

- Wood can break the ground (Earth).
- Earth can soak up Water, blocking its flow.
- Water can control Fire.
- Fire can melt Metal.
- Metal can chop Wood.

Overacting Cycle Cheng

The overacting (overwhelming) cycle (cheng) is an inbalance within the ke cycle, while following the ke cycle's direction. The grandparent element provides too much control over the grandchild and weakens the element. Each element excessivley restrains another beyond the normal extend. This usually occures when an element is in excess:

- Too much Wood overacts Fire.
- Too much Fire overacts Earth.
- Too much Earth overacts Metal.
- Too much Metal overacts Water.
- Too much Water overacts Wood.

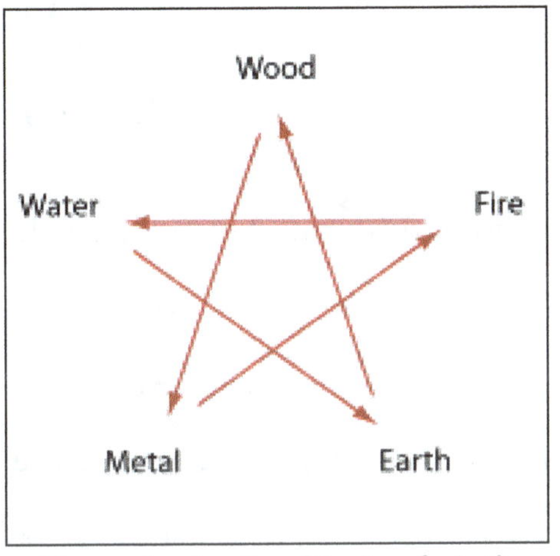

The weakening (insulting) cycle (wǔ).

The weakening (insulting) cycle: Grandchild insults or returnes the controlling force generated by the Grandparent.

The weakening cycle is an imbalance within the controlling cycle, where that, what is destroyed, enjures the destroyer. The imbalance follows along the opposite route of the ke cycle, each element can insult the one that normally restrains it. The reverse of the ke cycle normally occures when the balance is broken, especially when one element is insufficient.

Interpretation: Weakening cycle: Earth can bury Wood. Water washes away Earth. Fire enjures = evaporates Water.

- Too much Wood insults Metal.
- Too much Metal insults Fire.
- Too much Fire insults Water.
- Too much Water insults Earth.
- Too much Earth insults Wood.

Interrelation of the Cycles

Sheng and Ke cycle:

The Sheng and Ke cycle form a feedback system, which keeps the system/body/universe in balance. The Sheng and Ke cycle ensure that each element is connected with the other four elements.

Wood restrains Earth, but at the same time, the Earth promotes Metal, which than restrains the Wood. In this instance, Metal makes sure, that Wood does not restrain Earth too excessivley.

Ke and Wu cycle:

The Controling- Weakening cycle or Ke and Wu cycle represents a conflicting (fighting) aspect.

- Wood can break the ground (Earth), but Earth can bury Wood, too.
- Earth can absorb Water, but Water can cover the land (Earth).
- Water can extinguish Fire, but Fire might evaporate Water.
- Fire can melt Metal, but Metal might not melt before Fire is extinguished.
- Metal can cut Wood, but Metal might become dull before breaking Wood.

Wu and Cheng cycle:

If any of the elements are over abundant, they can disrupt the balance of the circle.

Characteristics and Associations of the Elements

Wood

Wood is the most human of the elements. It is the element of spring; the creative urge to achieve - which can turn to anger when frustrated. It is associated with the capacity to look forward, plan and make decisions, hence growth and expansion.

Wood energy is rising, expanding, and is the force of growth and flexibility, hence the colour associated with Wood is green and a rectangled shape.

This element represents all the activities of the body that are self regulating and/or function without conscious thought; i.e. digestion, respiration, heart beat and basic metabolism.

The liver (converting food into fuel which is then supplied to the muscles, tendons and ligaments) is associated to the Wood element as well as the gallbladder.

Wood represents as well the direction East, the planet Jupiter and is symbolized by an Azure Dragon.

Wood 'governs' the Chinese Zodiac signs Tiger, Rabbit and Dragon.

Fire

Fire is the element of heat, summer and enthusiasm; nature at its peak of growth, and warmth in human relationships.

Represented by the colour red and a pointed, triangled shape, Fire's motion is upward, hence is associated with dynamic, energetic, passionate, enterprising energies.

Fire is the symbolic of combustion and this represents the functions of the body that have reached the fleeting moment of maximum activity; indicating that decline is then inevitable.

The element is associated with the heart, the circulation system and is related to the tongue.

Fire represents the direction South, the planet Mars and is symbolized by a Vermilion Bird/(Red) Pheasant.

Fire 'governs' the Chinese Zodiac signs Snake, Horse and Sheep.

Earth

Earth is the element of harvest time, abundance, nourishment, fertility, and the mother to child relationship. This element is also regarded as central to balance and the place where energy becomes downward in movement, a change of seasons. It is the symbol of stability and being properly anchored.

Represented by the colour yellow and a square shape, Earth's motion is patient, reliable, logical, governed by service and duty to others, militaristic, stubborn, very energetic.

Earth is associated with the digestive system, stomach (middle of the body), the spleen and is related to the sense of taste.

Earth represents the direction Centre (Yellow Earth, China - Middle Land), the planet is Saturn, and is symbolized by the Yellow Dragon.

Earth 'governs' the Chinese Zodiac signs Dragon, Rat, and Ox. Earth is the central balance of the elements and can lend qualities to all 12 animals as well.

Metal

This category includes the Western idea of the air element. It is the force of gravity, the minerals within the earth, the patterns of the heavenly bodies and the powers of electrical conductivity and magnetism. Metal has structure, but it can also accept a new form when molten.

Metal energy is consolidating and with inward movement, like a flower closing its petals.

Represented by the colour white and round shapes, Metal's motion is determined, forceful, strong, unyielding, self- reliant, reserved and sophisticated.

The symbol of metal is one of a cutting and reforming action, but it is also regarded as a solidifying process, hence it is associated with Autumn.

Metal is associated with the lungs, respiratory system and is related to the nose.

Metal represents the direction West, the planet is Venus, and is symbolized by the White Tiger.

Metal 'governs' the Chinese Zodiac signs Monkey, Rooster and Dog.

Water

Water is the source of life on this planet. Water has the capacity to flow, infinitely yielding yet infinitely powerful, silent and still, awaiting, flexible, ever changing, a stored potential and often dangerous (flood's devastation) with the capacity also to nourish and cleanse.

Likewise it is the fluid (the main component of the body) which nourishes and maintains the health of every cell. Water corresponds to the skeletal and excretory system as well as to the vital fluids, i.e. blood, lymph, mucus, semen and fat and is related to the lung.

The kidney is especially linked to this element.

Represented by the colour black/blue and a wave like shape, Water's motion is downward, fluid, secretive, intuitive, compassionate, sensitive, gentle and creative.

Water is the ultimate yin; quiet, cold; representing the resting time of winter.

In human psychology the element governs the balance between fear or being exploited and the desire to dominate.

Water represents the direction North, the planet is Mercury, and is symbolized by the Black Tortoise. Water 'governs' the Chinese Zodiac signs Pig, Rat and Ox.

The characteristic of each phase (new yang through to full yin) is determined by what happens in the natural world during each associated season. One season after another plays its role in the cycle of the year by just doing what it does when it does it and then smoothly moves on to the next. It is the smooth and harmonious transition from one phase to another that is important, along with the balance between them.

THE FIVE ELEMENTS AND TASTE

The five elements theory is used as the basis of the universe and describes the way everything interacts, including human body systems. The five elements are: fire, wood, earth, metal and water. Our five major organs, namely heart, liver, spleen, lung and kidney, correspond to these five elements. Each of these organs is also linked to a flavour which can upset or help the function of that particular organ. These five flavours are: bitter, sour, sweet, pungent and salty.

The organs try to balance themselves through your diet. When an organ is upset, the body can send you signal by making you crave for a particular taste.

Heart Health

In Chinese medicine, excess heat at the heart could be damaging. When someone has excess heat, the body will show symptoms such as ulcers in the mouth, red face, emotional, heart palpitations, anxiety, insomnia and dreaminess. Chinese medicine practitioners believe that bitter taste can clear heat from the body, especially from the heart. Food like bitter gourd or bitter leafy greens all help with this condition.

Liver Health

Chinese medicine considers the liver and your mind/emotions to be closely connected to each other. When you are at peace, your liver is able to function properly. On the contrary, when your liver is upset, your body will experience a lot of emotional symptoms, such as being easily irritated. If there is qi (chi) stagnation at your liver, it could cause blood rise to the head and lead to headache, dizziness, or even insomnia. Chinese medicine suggests that eating sour food can calm your liver qi. You can also drink a little vinegar to unblock liver qi and help circulation.

Spleen

Unlike Western medicine, Chinese medicine considers the spleen as an important organ that dominates digestion, including functions of transformation, transportation and absorption of nutrients from food. In case of spleen disorder, the body might experience a lack of energy, bloating, irregular bowel movement, puffy arms and legs, etc. Deficiency of spleen qi often create craving for sweets because sweet flavours is believed to help tone spleen qi and energy. However, we do not recommend you to eat loads of sugar or sweet. Instead, go for the natural options and eat moderately, eg consider fruits, wholegrains, or sensible potion of natural sugar.

Lung

The lung is considered by Chinese medicine as the first defence of the body which fights against external pathogenic factors. When its function is impaired, we might have sneezing, cough, headache, sore throat, body aches, etc. Pungent flavours expel wind and cold pathogenic factors from the lung. Spice up a little by adding spring onion or ginger to your food especially during cold seasons.

Kidney

In Chinese medicine, kidney stores our body's original essence – inherited from our parents. Weak kidneys might lead to symptoms such as: lack of energy, low back pain, tired legs, poor memory, frequent urination especially at night time, early greying of hair, early menopause, impotence, etc. Salty flavours goes to the kidneys first. But be moderate with salt. Try black beans, walnuts, chestnuts, etc.

THE FIVE COLORS OF TCM

In traditional Chinese medicine (TCM) theory, according to the five elements (wood, fire, earth, metal, water) doctrine, the natural flavors (sour, bitter, sweet, acrid, salty), five colors of food (green, red, yellow, white, black) are linked with many properties of things. This shows the relationship between human and nature.

Humans live in between the universe and the earth; it, in the natural environment, is a part that makes up the material world, and should be fused with nature. There are colorful plants in nature, moisturized and growing under the sunlight and rain, providing food sources for human beings. The body's five internal organs and nature's five colors are closely linked.

Five colors that people are familiar with in daily life (green, red, yellow, white and black), works at different organs, and each one play a different role. Different colors of food are vastly different with their effectiveness on maintaining health. Different colors of food and their properties are not the same, and their effects are different too.

Green Nourishes Liver

Common green color food are those things like green beans, spinach (the most liver nourishing dish), broccoli, cucumber, gourd, celery, leek, green pepper, crowndaisy chrysanthemum, lettuce, cabbage, shepherd's purse (its name in Changsha: rapeseed, has heat-eliminating and antihypertension effects), Chinese cabbage, kidney beans, fresh kidney beans, water spinach (called Yong Choi and four voices in Changsha), Gynura cusimba, green amaranth, yin radish, pak choi, bitter gourd (eliminates heat at heart the most, and can secrete insulin), fruits and so on.

Red Nourishes the Heart

Common red-color food are red beans, sweet potatoes, carrots (the vegetable that protects the eyes the most, strengthen the spleen and protects the liver), red pepper, red dates, tomatoes, hawthorn, cedar, strawberry, etc.

Yellow Benefits the Spleen and Stomach

Common yellow-colored food are soybeans, burdock (best at eliminating spleen and stomach heat, you can make bones stew soup by combining with red and white radish), foot yam (best type of food in treatment of oral ulcers), barley, (sweet, mild and slightly cooling nature, can diuret and relieve swelling, strengthen the spleen and eliminate dampness, relieves muscular rheumatism, relieves heat and eliminates pus and other effects, commonly used as a diuretic and eliminate dampness medicine) leeks, pumpkin (to produce insulin, and treat diabetes related symptoms), apples, egg yolks, maize, corn, etc.

White Moistens Lungs

Common white color foods include white beans, winter melon, pear, white radish, white fungus, lotus root, lily, wild rice, rice, tofu, cauliflower, bamboo shoots, yam, jicama and so on.

Black Nourishes the Kidneys

Common black color food include black beans, black rice, black sesame, black fungus, walnut (not black, but it is a food that nourishes the kidneys), seaweed, kelp (also a food that moistens the lungs).

THE FIVE ELEMENTS OF THE CELL

Everything in the surrounding universe can be attributed into five elements. Human organs can be also linked to the five elements. Cells, the smallest unit of the human body, consist of cellular organelles as little organs.

Similar to how Greek philosophers have discussed the origin of all things in the universe, ancient philosophers in China also debated on how the origin and consequence of all things can be explained and cycled. They postulated that the universe is composed of five fundamental elements, and then they developed the theory of how the universe was created and it undergoes a cycling process. The 'five elements theory' not only defines the character of each element, but also emphasizes the mutual interaction and rotation of the elements under an interactive system.

The five elements or five phases, are orderly classified by five materials as follows: wood, fire, earth, metal, and water. Each element has its own literal and philosophical meaning. The wood-type is represented by a tree that grows straight and is abundantly spreading out. The fire-type is represented by a state of combustion that generates heat. It is likely that the earth-type will establish a foothold to newly change an outdated system. The metal-type is represented by the formation of hard crystal. Lastly, the water-type is represented by a stream that seems to run out of a solid melting. The attributions of each element in itself do not reveal their identities, but rather, reveal their color when under reciprocal interaction. There are two flows among the five elements, i.e., the mutual nourishment cycle and mutual restrain cycle which have organically positive or negative influences on each other.

Characteristics of the Five Elements

On the concept of five elements, everything, including forms of matter or even spirit, can be classified, and arranged into each of the five elements. Following the examples of the five phases, either the features or the appearance of all things can be used to categorize them into their own unique five phases. In terms of shape, the wood-type appears as long sticks, fire-type is symbolized by an inverted triangle, earth-type stands for wide ground, metal-type describes images of sharp edge, and water-type depicts the shape of a running stream. In addition to shapes, color is also applied to the five phases. Blue is a symbol of the wood-type; red is representative of the fire-type; yellow represents feeling comfortable and symbolizes soil, not only fostering but also supporting, the earth-type; white is the metal-type color of polished iron and silver; and black, which represents the ability to hide, is associated with the water-type.

Practical Application of the Five Elements

Doctors who practice traditional Chinese medicine (TCM) have put the five elements theory into practice, extending it to clinical practice as a form of five element acupuncture (FEA), which was introduced by a British acupuncturist, Dr J.R. Worsley. FEA is now a popular alternative treatment worldwide, including in Europe, Australia, and the United States. According to Dr Worsley, human bodies are composed of a combination of the five elements. A deficiency among the five elements are thought to cause illness. Thus, practitioners diagnose the deficient elements in the patients and treat illness by supplying the deficiency using FEA. There is also another FEA method, called Sa-Ahm acupuncture, in Korea. In Sa-Ahm acupuncture is applied on points called Five-Shu, which is five flows of qi divided by five elements at limb distal part below elbow or knee joint. Thus, even if there are differences among countries, the five elements theory can be practically applied to alternative medicine in the worldwide.

Five Elements and Human Organs

Prior to the introduction of functional organs under anatomical system, TCM had already established the human organic system, applying the above concept to human organs, consequently categorizing human organs according to the five elements, during China's Warring States Period. The classical book of Huangdi Neijing (also called the Inner Classic of the Yellow Emperor) connected each organ to five elements linked to natural phenomena, particularly weather; however, they lacked an explanation for causal relationships. Although it is still ideological theory, which is yet to be proven, TCM has developed this theory and applied it to functional organs and anatomical systems. TCM divides the human organic system into five organs, i.e., the liver, heart, pancreas (including spleen), lung, and kidney, which correspond to wood-, fire-, earth-, metal-, and water-type, respectively. The liver plays a role as the first of the five-phase cycle, supplying energy originating from glucose, fatty acids, and amino acids to the whole body, and even converting extra energy to glycogen storage, hormones, and proteins. Oriental medicine refers to the heart as the ruler of the human body, circulating blood, oxygen, nutrients, and waste. It is tied to the impression of furious flames. The pancreas is part of the digestive system. It produces insulin, which induces target cells to absorb glucose as an energy source that supplies the body. This function has been likened to that of the earth-type, which fosters crops. As the lid of the body, the lung is a respiratory organ for breathing, or the exchange of gas. The exchange of carbon dioxide and oxygen occurs in the lung, giving it metal-type attributes. Finally, the kidney plays a role in filtering the body's waste for removal and producing urine. Water, excreted from the kidney is reminiscent of the flow of a river; therefore, the kidney has a water-type attribute.

Five Elements and Cellular Organelles

The cell is functionally and structurally the smallest unit of the human body. By maintaining communication between extracellular and intracellular environments, cellular organelles perform the diverse functions required for cells to grow, divide, synthesize, package, and survive. The cellular organelles include the endoplasmic reticulum (ER), Golgi apparatus (GA), mitochondria, lysosome, and plasma membrane (PM), which envelopes the cell. Considering the concept of the fractal theory, i.e., typical self-similar patterns, cellular organelles may correspond to human organs. Thus, it then follows that cellular organelles can be classified as little organs. As explained above, since the five organs can be based on five phases, this can also be applied to the five cellular organelles. This means that human cellular organelles can also be orderly divided into five parts, where the ER, GA, lysosome (including vacuoles), mitochondria, and PM, correspond to wood-, fire-, earth-, metal-, and water-type, respectively. The ER is composed of three kinds of structural forms: cisternae, vesicles, and tubules. The ER can be structurally and functionally divided into the rough ER and smooth ER. The rough ER is involved in the synthesis of protein due to the many ribosomes lining its inside, while the smooth ER is involved in lipid, glycogen, and steroid synthesis. Thus, the main function of the ER is synthesis. Proteins that are synthesized at the ER are modified to direct them to their destinations. Like packaging in the post office, the GA acts as a central transport system and plays an important role in modifying, sorting, and packaging macromolecules for transportation. Each molecule cannot perform its functions until it has matured at the GA. Although each molecule completes its function at its destination, the by-products that are generated by metabolic processes need to be eventually recycled or removed. As the cellular digestive organelle, the lysosome contains hydrolase enzymes in its acidic compartment that can digest metabolic products or waste. In addition to the lysosome, vacuoles are also able to help process cellular waste. The function of vacuoles is to contain waste or water to isolate harmful contents from the cell. Like the lysosome, some vacuoles also have digestive function through maintaining an acidic internal pH and containing hydrolytic contents.

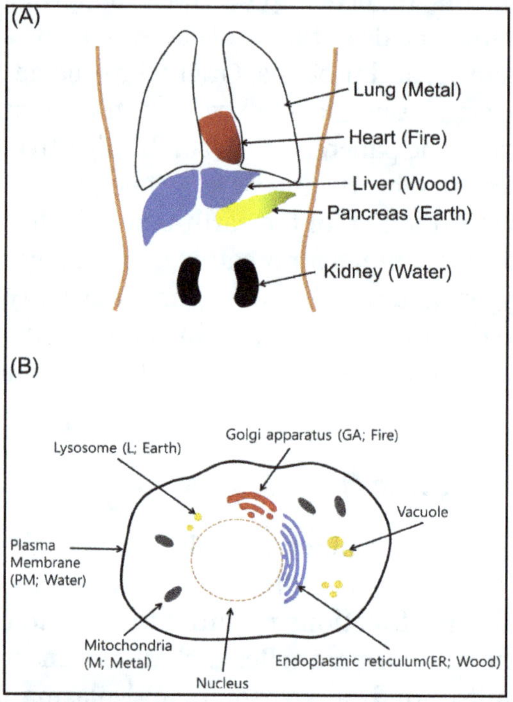

Diagram of human organs and cell structure.

Mitochondria provide the cell with energy (i.e., adenosine triphosphate) via oxidative respiratory phosphorylation, using oxygen, to carry out diverse metabolic tasks, such as apoptosis, calcium signaling, cellular metabolism, etc. Finally, the PM, acts as a selective filter, and separates the internal part of cell from the outer environment. It selectively transports ions, inorganic, and organic molecules through the membrane. The materials can be transported through the cell membrane by several mechanisms: 1) passive diffusion, 2) active transportation through transmembrane channels and transporters, 3) endocytosis, and 4) exocytosis. Thus, cellular organelles seem to have the attributes of little organs of the human body. Importantly, the nucleus, which is the control center of cell, could not be included in the five cellular organelles, because it corresponds to the brain, the control organ of the body, which is excluded from the list of five organs corresponding to the five elements. Overall, the ER, GA, lysosome, mitochondria, and PM, correspond to the liver, heart, pancreas, lung, and kidney. Certain aspects of oriental medicine, like the relationship between the organs and the five elements, may also be extended to the five elements. That is, based on the fractal theory, the five cellular organelles may be linked to the five elements that correspond to the five organs. The synthetic function of the ER makes itself have the characteristics of the wood-type, as does the liver. Similarly, the GA, lysosome (vacuole), mitochondria, and PM also correspond to fire-, earth-, metal-, and water-type, respectively.

Major human organs comprising the circulatory system like the lung and heart, digestive system like the liver and pancreas, and urinary system like the kidney (A). Representative cellular organelles include the nucleus, endoplasmic reticulum (ER), Golgi apparatus (GA), mitochondria (M), lysosome (L), vacuoles, and plasma membrane (PM) surrounding the cytosol of cells (B).

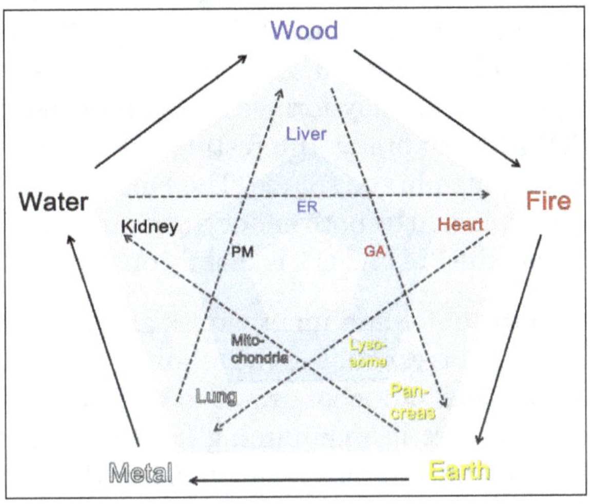

Diagram of linkage between cellular organelles extending to organs and five elements.

The clockwise rotation of five elements is order, circulates from the wood- to water-type. The human organs, which are connected to the five elements, also rotates along with them. The innermost pentagon indicates cellular organelles as microcosms of the five elements. Arrow-lines present mutual nourishment cycle, arrow-dashed lines indicate mutual restrain cycle. Pc indicates pancreas.

Relationships of Cellular Organelles in the Theory of Five Elements

As introduced above, there can be cycles of mutual nourishment and mutual restrain. The mutual nourishment cycle is the so-called win-win relationship that forms a circulation in the order of the ER, GA, lysosome, mitochondria, and PM. The mutual restrain cycle, however, is a balance of relationships that forms a circulation in the order of ER, lysosome, PM, GA, and mitochondria.

A representative example of the mutual nourishment cycle is the transportation of synthesized molecules, such as proteins and lipids, from the ER via the GA into the lysosome.

The mutually beneficial relationship between the lysosome and mitochondria is exemplified by the steady-state removal of reactive oxygen species formed in the process of mitochondrial respiration. The mitochondria-derived vesicles budding from the mitochondria can selectively carry reactive oxygen species to the lysosomes. The mitochondria supply the PM with energy to perform active transport across the membrane, in and out of various molecules through transporters. In relation to the circulation between the PM and ER, the PM, being tightly associated with the ER, can regulate Ca^{2+} signaling as well as organelle morphology through the interplay of the stromal-interaction molecule proteins.

In the mutual restrain cycle, the typical balance of processes is seen in the formation of autophagosomes, a double-membrane compartment that usually manifests under unfavorable starved conditions. This process involves mitochondria, the ER, GA, and lysosomes. Cells remove damaged molecules or waste products and organelles through the process of autophagy. The core of this process is the formation of the autophagosome, which eventually fuses with lysosomes, degrading its contents and forming the autolysosome. Autophagosomes are initially formed at ER-mitochondria contact sites, i.e., mitochondria-associated ER membrane. Interestingly, the GA is known to be involved in autophagy as a potential membrane source. The balanced relationship between the lysosome and PM can be explained by both endocytosis and exocytosis, whereas the balanced relationship between the PM and GA is mainly observed in exocytosis.

As explained above, both the outer and inner circles are linked to the five elements in an intriguing manner, which corresponds to the relationships of the five cellular organelles (i.e., the ER, GA, lysosome, mitochondria, and PM). These relationships between the organelles have central roles in maintaining homeostasis in both intra- and extra-cellular environments and metabolism, which is like the mutual nourishment and restrain cycles of the five elements.

Perspective Study of Cellular Organelles on the Theory of Five Elements

It may be too obvious that the latest theories in biology have not taken into account the idea of conceptual and reciprocal of five elements theory, as it has evolved through the interpretation of results through experimental and analytical methods. Thus, efforts to identify the mutual nourishment or restrain cycle between microscopic cellular organelles in a systematical and experimental manner have not been considered. However, since stem cell research has recently become more prominent, pluripotent stem cells might provide a resource to prove the cellular five elements, with the hypothesis that the interaction between cellular organelles, or mutual nourishment or restrain of cellular organelles, will also be experimentally verified in terms of cell type. For example, in the case of pluripotent stem cells, there is a difference in the number of mitochondria before and after differentiation which is a simple example showing that the role of cell organelles can change with different cell types. In addition, cancer cells can produce energy by the Warburg effect by mitochondrial respiration defects due to mitochondria abnormalities. Although mitochondrial metabolism can play an important role in chemotherapy, other organelles such as ER (mutual nourishment of mitochondria) and GA (mutual restrain of that) can also be targeted by chemotherapy. Thus, mitochondria can be considered to either be a part of the mutual nourishment cycle or restrain cycle.

THE IMBALANCE OF THE FIVE ELEMENTS

The Five Elements, or Five Phases, are aspects of Qi. These are Wood, Fire, Earth, Metal, and Water. In the poetic language of the Five Elements, health is a harmonious balance of all the elements. The Qi of the elements waxes and wanes in daily and seasonal cycles. Each one of us is a unique and characteristic blend of the influences of all the elements.

Wood Imbalance

When the wood Qi is weak, people can be indecisive, without strong direction in life, and stuck. They may be constrained emotionally, unable to express anger. When the Liver Qi is congested or stagnant, people can be arrogant, over controlling, and have angry dispositions. They may have a tendency to be workaholics or have addictive personalities, including the possibility of abusing drugs and alcohol. They may have digestive problems like bloating, gas, alternating constipation and diarrhea.

When Liver Qi is imbalanced, hot and spicy foods may cause too much heat. Sour and bitter flavors are said to benefit the Liver meridian. Excessive frustration and irritation can be especially difficult when the Liver meridian is out of balance. Physical exercise and reading can help restore balance. The fall is a vulnerable time, as well as the winds of March, and extremely hot weather.

Common signs of Liver meridian stress include dry, brittle, thickened nails and pain just below the ribs. Common illnesses include migraines, eye problems, and sinus problems. The Liver meridian circles the genitals, and rashes and discharges are associated with its imbalance, as well as hernias. For women, menstrual problems are common including PMS, painful periods, and heavy bleeding. Uterine fibroids may be related to imbalance of the Liver meridian as well. The Liver and Gallbladder meridian pathways traverse the top and sides of the head, the most common sites for migraine headaches.

The Qi of the Wood element flourishes in the spring when plants are sprouting new growth; and the color of this element is green.

Earth Imbalance

When people have weak Earth Qi, they can be worriers and meddlers. They are prone to pensiveness. They may overwork, especially in studying or other intellectual work.

They are vulnerable to digestive problems and diarrhea. They may gain weight easily and lose it with difficulty. Their bodies have a tendency to make excessive mucus, and they may suffer from cloudy thinking, muzzy-headedness, and a lack of clarity.

Those with weak Earth Qi often feel better when they limit cold, raw foods and dairy products. They should eat warming foods and grains to stay well grounded. They may crave sweets. The sweet taste can be satisfied by eating sweet grains, vegetables, and fruits rather than processed sugars.

Common illnesses include: fatigue, diarrhea, gas & bloating, food allergies & sensitivities, eating disorders, heartburn, and canker sores. Excessive mucus may collect in the lungs or in the sinuses. In women, menstrual problems may include either excessively light or heavy periods.

The Qi of the earth element flourishes in Indian Summer, those golden moments of fullness before the waning of the light. The earth color is yellow, like the sun, and the ripened crops, and the root vegetables. Sitting meditation is said to strengthen the earth element.

Metal Imbalance

A person with Metal Qi imbalance may be grief-stricken, steeped in sadness. They may be overly critical. They may have trouble letting go. When the Metal energy is weak, there can be illnesses of the lungs – asthma, allergies, frequent colds. The Lung meridian rules the skin, so rashes, eczema, and problems with sweating can be related to Metal imbalance. The Large Intestine meridian can be affected by chronic constipation or diarrhea, or other bowel diseases.

The Metal energy peaks in the fall. In the cool, crisp, clean air of autumn, metal people feel they can accomplish anything. The color of Metal is white, and people strongly influenced by the Metal Qi may have pale complexions.

Water Imbalance

When the Kidney Qi is weak, there can be problems with water metabolism, urination, fertility, or sexuality. This person could be anxious, fearful, and withdrawn, and in more severe cases, phobic.

Kidney Qi declines with aging. There may be diminished hearing or ringing in the ears. In menopause, the Kidney yin declines, which is associated with classic signs of heat and dryness – hot flashes, night sweats, dry skin and mucous membranes. Kidney yang weakness is associated with cold – cold extremities, cold back and belly, declining sexual vigor, urinary frequency or incontinence.

The color of the Kidney is black, like the night, or like black ice. When the Kidney Qi starts to weaken, dark circles or pouches appear under the eyes. The Kidney Qi rules in the winter, a time when living things are contracted with cold. Like a seed deep in the cold ground, Qi is dormant, waiting for the time to sprout.

References

- Five-elements, Chinese-Customs, oneworld: nationsonline.org, Retrieved 8 June, 2020
- The-five-flavours-and-the-five-organs-from-tcms-perspective: one-organic.com, Retrieved 5 March, 2020
- 11-the-five-colors-of-tcm, item: imperialtcm.com, Retrieved 1 August, 2020
- PMC5741387, pmc: ncbi.nlm.nih.gov, Retrieved 11 January, 2020
- Tradition: acupuncture-online.com, Retrieved 12 July, 2020

The Concept of Illness

CHAPTER 5

In traditional Chinese medicine, illness is an imbalance of qi and Yin Yang rather than a purely physical phenomenon. It follows eight principles of diagnosis that are Yin and Yang, interior, exterior, heat, cold, deficiency and excess. The topics elaborated in this chapter will help in gaining a better perspective about the related concepts of illness and diagnosis in traditioanl Chinese medicine.

In Traditional Chinese Medicine (TCM) Internal causes were those which did not arise from what we might call catching a bug or a virus.

In designing a treatment, the patient's symptoms were and are more important than the original cause of the disease. However, understanding the cause often leads to better prognosis and treatment, so they are connected.

Constitution

Inherited factors can play a huge part in an individual's health. However, even if someone has a weak constitution, with forethought and self-discipline he may live much longer and more healthily than someone with a robust constitution who squanders his health through poor lifestyle choices.

Specifically, the health we inherit is said to depend on:

- Each of the parents' (and grandparents') general health.
- The parents' health at or leading up to the moment of conception.
- The mother's health during pregnancy.

One should also consider the age of the parents when the child was conceived. Sperm from an older father may be less virile and the ovum from an older mother less capable. If the mother is older at conception, her reserves of Kidney qi may be reduced with less available for a healthy pregnancy and child. Nowadays mothers have heard about the ill-effects of smoking and alcohol during pregnancy.

For example, Australian scientists discovered considerable adverse changes in the structure of babies' heads when their mothers consistently drank alcohol during pregnancy.

Trauma

The effects of trauma are usually immediately noticeable. However, trauma, for instance a back injury, from which the individual fully recovered in youth, may produce symptoms years later when the individual is exposed to external pathogenic factors that his aging vitality is no longer able to combat. Then, although the trauma occurred long before, it still counts as one of the internal causes of disease.

Trauma usually cause conditions of Blood Stasis.

Over-exertion and Over-work

- Over-exertion is relative to the constitution of the individual.
- A trained world-class athlete is capable of continued exertion that would be hardly imaginable for a normal individual, yet even such an athlete can, and not infrequently does, over-exert himself.
- This leads to a period of lowered energy and need to rest to recuperate.
- Usually this is thrust on the athlete by injury. It can also occur where an ageing athlete persists in exertion levels that were appropriate only when younger.
- Over-exertion as one of the internal causes of disease includes working too hard, for too long, or working without proper rest. It can include over-exertion of a particular part of the anatomy (e.g. vision if the individual works too long at a computer; repetitive strain injury where someone repeats a particular movement too often).
- Overwork leads to yin deficiency, mainly of Kidney yin, but potentially also of Liver Yin.
- Repetitive strain injury leads to Blood Stasis.
- Over-use of the eyes leads to deficiency of Liver Blood.
- These over-exertion internal causes of disease are often hard to accept when they occur. People understandably believe that they are living busy lives and must work hard.
- This doesn't alter the potential for long-term problems.

Emotions

Traditionally there are seven emotions that, unresolved, can be major internal causes of disease if they persist or are over-indulged in.

A slightly expanded list of these gives:

- Unrestrained or inappropriate joy, laughter (what we might call hysterical over-excitement): Affects the Heart.

- Worrying, over-thinking, obsession: Affects mainly the Spleen.
- Grief, sadness, worry: Mainly affects the Lungs.
- Sadness also affects the Heart.
- Fear, deep anxiety: Affects the Kidney.
- Anger, frustration: Affects the Liver.
- Shock affects the Heart and the Kidneys.

However, the connections between emotion and Organ (or Zang-fu) should not be taken too rigidly. Any of the Organs may be affected by any emotion. So prolonged Fear could affect not just the Kidneys but also the Liver, leading to a lack of nerve or of courage. All emotions have an effect on the Heart.

Any emotion, if one of the internal causes of disease, impairs the circulation of qi and blood. In particular it affects the direction of flow of qi.

- Anger makes qi rise: This we see in the face, the eyes, the complexion, the tension in the shoulders and neck, the grinding of teeth, the biting of nails or lips and so on.
- Joy slows down the movement of Qi: As when someone is speechless from joy or surprise.
- Sadness dissolves qi: As when, feeling hopeless sadness we find we lack energy to do anything: we sink, dejected.
- Over-thinking ties up (knots up) qi: Someone who is thinking about something too much can't make up their minds about it.
- Fear descends qi: Involuntarily our knees give way or we defecate or urinate.
- Shock scatters qi: We shake, we sweat, we go pale, we can't stand, our pulse races uncontrolled.

As internal causes of disease, severe emotional trauma can have lifelong effects on health, even after the individual has made serious attempts to accept the trauma and its consequences.

Excessive Sexual Activity

As one of the internal causes of disease, this is the least acceptable to many people nowadays - at least in developed countries. Perhaps for the ancient Chinese who lived in uncertain times, in conditions of hygiene we would find unacceptable, with food sources that were often unreliable, guarding their 'essence-qi' was more vital than now.

But even now, many people worldwide live in conditions not so different to the ancient Chinese.

On the other hand, many people living in the developed world believe that there is no limit to what they can have health-wise, because their nationalised health service is free, with abundant resources to repair any damage they do to themselves. Increasingly, women nowadays are demanding abortions if they don't like the sex or probable astrological birth sign of their foetus.

An abortion, in Chinese medicine, can seriously upset the flow of qi and Blood on which the woman's future health depends: it is a surgical procedure which may not only cause Blood Stasis but can drain the woman's Kidney essence.

In any case, 'Excessive Sexual Activity' has to be understood in relation to age and health of the individual. People in poor health should indulge less often. It is said that a rough estimate of how often a man should ejaculate is to divide his age by 5, giving the number of days between ejaculations. For instance, a 30 year old should, according to this recommendation, not ejaculate more often than once every 6 days. Clearly, however, much depends on the man's health, commitments and lifestyle. Stress of any kind may impair his ability and drain his energy but sometimes for a healthy man under stress, ejaculation can be cathartic.

Sexual activity for men is easy to describe: it means sperm ejaculation, which in Chinese Medicine is said to use up Kidney Essence. For women, the question of what excessive sexual activity means is less clear. Normal orgasm for women doesn't use Kidney essence.

However, any sexual activity that is exhausting must be considered, including, for some, having too many babies close together, without proper recovery between them. Blood loss from the womb that is uncontrolled would have a similar effect, such as in menorrhagia.

Abstention from sex when there is desire may also, long-term, harm the individual. What is called Minister Fire ascends during sexual desire and orgasm sends it down. If no orgasm then occurs, it may remain ascended and, eventually impair Heart qi or cause Heart Fire. Tantric traditions teach that non ejaculating during sex means that no Kidney essence is used up and can, so long as there is periodical ejaculation, enhance sexual experience. When in poor health, or recuperating from illness, men should indulge much less in orgasm with ejaculation.

Diet

- What we eat and how we eat it have major long-term repercussions on our health and can be major internal causes of disease.
- There is growing evidence for the benefits of choosing food that is nutritious,

fresh, high in vegetables, olive and essential oils, low in meat, alcohol, sugar and grains.

- Eat food when sitting, unhurried and not otherwise engaged; chew well; leave time for digestion after meals. Eat regularly, don't skip meals and don't eat too close to bedtime or late in the evening.
- Chinese medicine stresses that the foods we eat should be appropriate for our metabolism; that we should avoid too much raw and cold or iced food and drink, even if feeling well, let alone if ill.
- The same goes for too much very spicy, dairy and greasy food.
- Avoid both over- and under-eating.
- Short-term deviations from healthy eating probably don't matter. However, a period of months or years with a bad diet can have life-long effects.

Parasites

- Parasites can be one of the internal causes of disease but this is less common nowadays in developed countries.
- Parasites use the body's supplies of Qi and Blood, so drain Spleen qi and often cause symptoms of Dampness and Heat which themselves favour production of more parasites.
- They arise mainly from poor hygiene and diet, though in some countries parasites enter via the eyes, the ureter, anus or vagina, for example when swimming in infested water.
- Any diet that weakens the Spleen energy encourages conditions that harbour parasites.

EMOTIONAL IMBALANCE

In traditional Chinese medicine, emotions and physical health are intimately connected. Sadness, nervous tension and anger, worry, fear, and overwork are each associated with a particular organ in the body. For example, irritability and inappropriate anger can affect the liver and result in menstrual pain, headache, redness of the face and eyes, dizziness and dry mouth.

A diagnosis in traditional Chinese medicine is highly individualized. Once an organ system is identified, the unique symptoms of the patient determine the practitioner's treatment approach.

Using the liver again as an example, breast distension, menstrual pain, and irritability during menses are treated with certain herbs and acupuncture points. Headaches, dizziness, and inappropriate anger with redness of the face point to a different type of liver pattern and is treated in a different way.

What does the liver have to do with migraines? Organ systems in the traditional Asian sense may include the Western medical-physiological function, but are also part of a holistic body system. The liver, for example, ensures that energy and blood flow smoothly throughout the body. It also regulates bile secretion, stores blood, and is connected with the tendons, nails, and eyes.

By understanding these connections, we can see how an eye disorder such as conjunctivitis might be due to an imbalance in the liver, or excess menstrual flow may be due to dysfunction in the liver's blood-storing ability. Besides emotions, other factors such as dietary, environmental, lifestyle, and hereditary factors also contribute to the development of imbalances.

Spleen

- Emotions: Worry, dwelling or focusing too much on a particular topic, excessive mental work.
- Spleen Function: Food digestion and nutrient absorption. Helps in the formation of blood and energy. Keeps blood in the blood vessels. Connected with muscles, mouth, and lips. Involved in thinking, studying, and memory.
- Symptoms of Spleen Imbalance: Tired, loss of appetite, mucus discharge, poor digestion, abdominal distension, loose stools or diarrhea. Weak muscles, pale lips. Bruising, excess menstrual blood flow, and other bleeding disorders.
- Spleen Conditions: Spleen Qi Deficiency, Spleen Qi Descending, Spleen Yang Deficiency.

Lung

- Emotions: grief, sadness, detached.
- Lung Function: Respiration. Forms energy from air, and helps to distribute it throughout the body. Works with the kidney to regulate water metabolism. Important in the immune system and resistance to viruses and bacteria. Regulates sweat glands and body hair, and provides moisture to the skin.
- Symptoms of Lung Imbalance: Shortness of breath and shallow breathing, sweating, fatigue, cough, frequent cold and flu, allergies, asthma, and other lung conditions. Dry skin. Depression and crying.

- Lung Conditions: Lung Qi Deficiency, Lung Yin Deficiency, and Cold Damp Obstructing the Lungs.

Liver

- Emotions: Anger, resentment, frustration, irritability, bitterness, "flying off the handle".
- Liver Function: Involved in the smooth flow of energy and blood throughout the body. Regulates bile secretion, stores blood, and is connected with the tendons, nails, and eyes.
- Symptoms of Liver Imbalance: Breast distension, menstrual pain, headache, irritability, inappropriate anger, dizziness, dry, red eyes and other eye conditions, tendonitis.
- Liver Conditions: Liver Qi Stagnation, Liver Fire.

Heart

- Emotions: Lack of enthusiasm and vitality, mental restlessness, depression, insomnia, despair.
- Heart Function: Regulates the heart and blood vessels. Responsible for even and regular pulse. Influences vitality and spirit. Connected with the tongue, complexion, and arteries.
- Symptoms of Heart Imbalance: Insomnia, heart palpitations and irregular heartbeat, excessive dreaming, poor long-term memory, psychological disorders.
- Heart Conditions: Heart Yin and Heart Fire.

Kidney

- Emotions: Fearful, weak willpower, insecure, aloof, isolated.
- Kidney Function: Key organ for sustaining life. Responsible for reproduction, growth and development, and maturation. Involved with lungs in water metabolism and respiration. Connected with bones, teeth, ears, and head hair.
- Symptoms of Kidney Imbalance: Frequent urination, urinary incontinence, night sweats, dry mouth, poor short-term memory, low back pain, ringing in the ears, hearing loss, and other ear conditions. Premature gray hair, hair loss, and osteoporosis.
- Kidney Conditions: Kidney Yin Deficiency and Kidney Yang Deficiency.

Using TCM

Since symptoms of these TCM syndromes in alternative medicine may be linked to a number of medical conditions, it's important to consult your physician if you have any health concerns. Self-treating a health condition and avoiding or delaying standard care may have serious consequences.

DIAGNOSIS IN TRADITIONAL CHINESE MEDICINE

Diagnosis in traditional Chinese medicine may appear to be simply a grouping of symptoms, but the elegance of Chinese medicine is that a diagnosis automatically indicates a treatment strategy.

For example, a woman experiencing menopause may have hot flashes, night sweats, thirst, and irritability; this group of symptoms leads to a diagnosis of kidney yin deficiency with heat. This diagnosis immediately points to the indicated therapy: Tonify kidney yin and clear deficiency heat. Since standard formulas are available for this pattern, such as Rehmannia Teapills, an accurate diagnosis enables a practitioner to prescribe a treatment that has been proved safe and effective for thousands of years.

A practitioner can obtain all of the information needed to diagnose disease through inquiry and external observation. The four basic categories of diagnostic observation are looking, listening and smelling, asking, and touching. Simply by employing these four areas of investigation, traditional practitioners can accurately assess physical and emotional imbalances of the internal organs and reestablish harmony.

It is important to remember that diagnostic indicators are always viewed holistically – that is, in total and in relation to the whole person. For example, fatigue is a symptom of qi or blood deficiency, but fatigue is also a symptom in a case of wind cold. If a person with wind cold was mistakenly diagnosed with qi deficiency, he might be given ginseng, a strong tonic that would make the symptoms much worse.

A careful practitioner would note that the person's pulse was strong and floating, a sign of wind cold, while a person with qi deficiency would have a deep and weak pulse. While it is necessary to learn the individual diagnostic patterns, it is crucial to remember that any sign or symptom must be viewed in relation to the whole person.

EIGHT PRINCIPLES OF DIAGNOSIS

Yin and Yang Theory

The theory of yin and yang is the most fundamental concept of traditional Chinese medicine. One of the major beliefs of TCM is that all things in the universe are either yin or yang. However, there are no absolutes: nothing is ever all yin or all yang, but a balance between the two forces. For example, when day changes into night, it is an example of a yang object changing into a yin object; when winter turns into spring; it is considered a changing from yin to yang. These forces are opposite and yet complementary, and share an interdependent relationship without yin, there would be no yang, and without yang, no yin.

Yang is generally associated with items or concepts that are bright, warm, and in motion. Yin is generally associated with objects or ideas that are dark, still and cold. Any given frame of reference can be divided into opposite factors, i.e. a yin side and a yang side. For instance, a human body can be divided into exterior and interior sections; the temperature can be divided into hot or cold; time can be divided into day or night; animals can divided into hot-blooded or cold-blooded, and so on.

The following are some of the more well-known examples of yin and yang:

Yin	Yang
Female	Male
Night	Day
Moist	Dry
Cold	Hot
Winter	Summer
Death	Birth
Small	Large
Solid	Hollow

The Yin-Yang Symbol

The yin-yang symbol is a representation of the philosophy of traditional Chinese medicine. The symbol consists of a circle, divided by a curved line into a black (yin) and white (yang) side. The curve symbolizes the constant change of balance between yin and yang. Each side contains a small circle of the opposite color. This demonstrates the belief that nothing is never really all yin or all yang; there is some of yang in yin, and vice-versa.

Applying Yin and Yang to Chinese Medicine

Each organ in the body has an element of yin and yang within it. Some organs, such as the liver, are predominantly yang; others, such as the kidneys, are yin. Even though an organ may be predominantly yin or yang in nature, the balance of yin and yang is maintained throughout the body, because the sum total of yin and yang will be in balance.

It is important to note that the body is not always in an exact balance of yin and yang. Even when the body is healthy, there may be subtle shifts from one state to the other. When a person gets angry, for instance, the yang state may dominate; when that person has calmed down and resumed to a peaceful state, yin may become dominant.

In traditional Chinese medicine, illness is believed to be caused by an imbalance of yin and yang in the body. In an excess of yin, the yang qi would be damaged, leading to the development of a cold disease. Excess of yang will likewise damage yin qi and lead to a heat disease being developed.

Basic treatment of these diseases is aimed at replenishing depleted yin or yang, and it is through this process that the balance of yin and yang is re-established. Traditional Chinese medicine practitioners attempt to determine the exact nature of the imbalance, then correct it through a variety of approaches, including acupuncture, herbal remedies, exercise, and changes in diet and lifestyle. As the balance is restored in the body, so is the person's health.

Exterior and Interior

Exterior and interior determine the severity of a disease and the affected body part. If a disease occurs in the body surface, muscles, or meridians, it is usually regarded as an exterior type (affected superficial portion of the body) and unlikely to be serious. If a disease occurs in the organs, blood, qi (vital energy) and bone marrow, it is regarded as an interior type and likely to be relatively serious. The exterior and interior principles are especially important for diagnosing exogenous diseases. Since their causal factors are originated from outside the body, they tend to have typical course of development, such as from outer to inner part of body, from superficial to deep regions, and even aggravated progressively, therefore physicians are able to evaluate and predict the clinical stage of patients according to the two principles.

Syndromes of Exterior Type

This refers to conditions resulting from an invasion of exogenous pathogens that enter through the mouth, nose or body surface, and affect the superficial portion of the body. The conditions are marked by sudden onset, relative gentle and short duration, that typically seen in early stage of feverish conditions. The clinical features of exterior type are fever, aversion to wind blowing, chills, headache, general aches, a thin tongue coating and a floating pulse. Other accompanying symptoms are nasal congestion, runny nose, sneezing, itchy and sore throat, and coughing.

Syndromes of Interior Type

This refers to pathological changes deep inside the body that involves the organs, bone marrow, qi or blood. Besides exogenous pathogens, factors like mental distress, improper diet and physical strain also lead to this type. Unlike the exterior type, clinical features of interior syndromes vary from person to person, and are mainly associated with organ dysfunctions, which have discussed in the section of Syndromes Differentiation According to Organs (zang-fu). Interior syndromes tend to be relative serious and longer course of disease. The clinical features of interior type are marked by NO aversion to wind and chills, never show a floating pulse, and there are usually tongue and the coating changes.

Disease symptoms usually change over time, and therefore, so can the type of syndrome a person experiences. Exterior and interior syndromes can mutually interchange, and even coexist such as simultaneous exterior and interior type or half exterior-half interior type.

Based on the clinical features, an exterior or interior syndrome is further linked with other principles.

	Exterior syndrome	Interior syndrome
Cold type	Fever, chills, headache, body aching, nasal congestion, sweating or lack of sweating, floating and tense pulse, thin white tongue coating.	Chills, cold limbs, pale complexion, lack of thirst or preference for hot drinks, nausea, vomiting, abdominal pain, diarrhea, clear profuse urine, deep and slow pulse, white and glossy tongue coating.
Heat type	Fever, slight aversion to wind and chills, sweating, slight thirst, sore throat, floating and rapid pulse, a red tongue.	High fever, sweating, thirst that preference for cold drinks, irritability, restlessness, red face, chapped lips, abdominal distention, constipation, yellow scanty urine, red tongue with yellow and dry coating, surging and rapid pulse, or deep and rapid pulse.
Deficiency (xu) type	Aversion to wind, sweating, floating and slow and forceless pulse. The tongue body is slightly bulky.	Feeble voice, breath shortness, apathy, general weakness, poor appetite, palpitation, dizziness, abdominal pain that feel alleviated when pressed, incontinence, deep and weak pulse, the tongue is pale and bulky and tender with white coating.
Excess (shi) type	Chills, fever, lack of sweating, headache, body aching, floating and tense pulse, or floating and forceful pulse, white tongue coating.	Coarse breathing, irritability, fullness in chest, abdominal distention and pain that become worse when pressed, constipation, yellow scanty urine, sweating in the palms and soles, deep and excess pulse, a rough and dry tongue with thick coating..

Cold

The cold pathogenic factor is considered a yin evil qi. Its nature is to slow movement down, causing tightness, contraction, stagnation, and impaired circulation. When it is an external pathogenic factor, cold can attack the skin, muscles, and lungs. When it is an internal pathogenic factor, cold can cause an impairment in the normal functions of the spleen, stomach, and kidneys.

Syndromes of Cold

Wind Cold: In combination with the pathogenic factor of wind, cold attacks the exterior of the body and the lungs, causing chills, lack of sweating, occipital headache (pain at the base of the skull), upper body aches, tight shoulders and neck, and a congested nose. The influence of wind causes the symptoms to appear suddenly and affect the upper body, while cold causes the muscles to contract, causing the stiffness and pain. Nasal secretions are clear – another sign of cold. The treatment principle is to repel the wind and disperse the cold with warm diaphoretic herbs, acupuncture, and moxibustion.

Obstruction Due to Cold: Traditionally known as cold bi (blockage) pain, this condition typically takes the form of body aches or joint pain that is relieved by warmth. The most common Western diagnosis for this pattern is arthritis. Since the syndrome is caused by cold, the joint may actually feel cold to the touch, and the pain typically gets worse in cold weather. The Chinese treatment principle is to increase circulation and warm the acupuncture meridians through which qi and blood circulate by means of moxibustion, acupuncture, and herbs.

Cold Attacking the Spleen and Stomach: In this externally caused disorder, cold causes digestive symptoms such as abdominal pain, clear vomit, and watery diarrhea. Although it usually accompanies an externally contracted cold or stomach bacteria or virus (what we commonly refer to as stomach "flu"), this syndrome can also be caused by eating cold foods such as ice cream.

Cold Congealing the Liver Meridian: The liver meridian passes through the genital area, and this condition is a manifestation of cold in that meridian. Symptoms include testicular pain or shrinking and hernia pain. Moxibustion, acupuncture, and herbs can effectively correct this imbalance in a short time.

Spleen Yang Deficiency: If a person has an underlying deficiency of spleen yang (deficiency in energy and heat needed in order to digest food), cold can severely impair digestive function. Symptoms of spleen yang deficiency include watery stools with undigested food, cold extremities, edema, and a slow pulse. When a person with this underlying deficiency is also affected by external cold pathogens, the imbalance is especially difficult to eliminate.

Treatment first expels the cold pathogenic factor. Then it tonifies the yang aspect of the spleen and kidneys to bring about a long-term increase in the body's basic metabolism, or its ability to maintain the heat needed for proper digestion, which is known in traditional Chinese medicine as life-gate (metabolic) fire. Spleen yang deficiency is treated with moxibustion and warming herbs that tonify spleen yang.

Kidney Yang Deficiency: Since the kidneys are the source of yang metabolic fire for the entire body, a deficiency in kidney yang can make the individual especially prone to cold. The symptoms of kidney yang deficiency include an inability to stay warm, cold extremities, low sex drive, frequent urination, edema (fluid retention), and pain in the low back. The yang deficiency can be corrected with long-term application of moxibustion and consumption of herbs that tonify kidney yang, thereby increasing metabolic fire.

Heat

Inflammation, a normal adaptive response of the organism to challenge, is important for survival. But it's run amok today, spurring an epidemic of chronic inflammatory conditions that morph into maladies as diverse as heart disease, diabetes, dementia, allergies, ADHD, reflux, and inflammatory bowel disorders.

From the perspective of Chinese medicine, modern life generates excess Heat. In Western terms, this is a result of sympathetic overdrive—too much cortisol and adrenalin—that set the stage for inflammation.

The solution in Chinese medicine is to restore the inner terrain, supporting host resilience. By nourishing the yin (moisture, blood), the overstimulation that produces excess yang (heat) is tempered.

Whenever the homeodynamic balance in the body is overtaxed, there's an up-regulating metabolic process that raises internal temperature. This is the progenitor of inflammation. The fight or flight response raises blood pressure, elevates heart rate, and releases glucose into the blood stream. When stress becomes chronic, these reaction patterns become entrenched.

Chinese medicine explains that prolonged stress breeds congestion–stagnation of qi and blood and the formation of phlegm. This disturbs circulation (hot head and trunk and cold limbs). A general increase in metabolic heat ensues, drying secretions, making them sticky and difficult to discharge.

The concept of phlegm explains a primary cause of illness and poor health. Degradation of the quality, viscosity, and distribution of body secretions interferes with three critical functions: circulation, breathing, and cognition.

When phlegm and heat accumulate, they transform into a fog-like mist that rises upward, obstructing the organs of perception (eyes, ears, nose, mouth, tongue). "Phlegm Heat misting the Mind" translates as an impaired ability to see, hear and think clearly, to learn, or make intelligent choices.

Acupuncture and herbal medicine clear heat and phlegm, replenish healthy substances (blood, moisture, essence), and thereby reduce stress and inflammation. Physiological and psychological equilibrium are restored, rebooting the body's ability to cope with challenges. Whether you have anxiety, high cholesterol, sinusitis, cough, headache, or an irritable bowel.

Here are ways in which some key body systems react:

- Nervous System: when stressed, physically or psychologically, the body suddenly shifts its energy resources to fighting off the perceived threat. In what is known as the "fight or flight" response, the sympathetic nervous system signals the adrenal glands to release adrenaline and cortisol. These hormones make the heart beat faster, raise blood pressure, change the digestive process and boost glucose levels in the bloodstream. Once the crisis passes, body systems usually return to normal.
- Musculoskeletal System: Under stress, muscles tense up. The contraction of muscles for extended periods can trigger tension headaches, migraines and various musculoskeletal conditions.
- Respiratory System: Stress can make you breathe harder and cause rapid breathing – or hyperventilation – which can bring on panic attacks in some people.
- Cardiovascular System: Acute stress, stress that is momentary, such as being stuck in traffic, causes an increase in heart rate and stronger contraction of the heart muscle. Blood vessels that direct blood to the large muscles and to the heart dilate, increasing the amount of blood pumped to these parts of the body. Repeated episodes of acute stress can cause inflammation in the coronary arteries, thought to lead to heart attack.
- Endocrine System.
- Adrenal glands: when the body is stressed, the brain sends signals from the hypothalamus, causing the adrenal cortex to produce cortisol and the adrenal medulla to produce epinephrine – sometimes called the "stress hormones".
- Liver: When cortisol and epinephrine are released, the liver produces more glucose, a blood sugar that would give you energy for "fight or flight" in an emergency
- Gastrointestinal System.
- Esophagus: Stress may prompt you to eat much more or much less than you usually do. If you eat more or different foods or increase your use of tobacco or alcohol, you may experience heartburn or acid reflux.

- Stomach: Your stomach can react with "butterflies" or even nausea or pain. You may vomit if the stress is severe enough. Bowels – Stress can affect digestion and which nutrients your intestines absorb. It can also affect how quickly food moves through your body. You may find that you have either diarrhea or constipation
- Reproductive System: In men, excess amounts of cortisol, produced under stress, can affect the normal functioning of the reproductive system. Chronic stress can impair testosterone and sperm production and cause impotence. In women, stress can cause absent or irregular menstrual cycles or more painful periods. It can also reduce sexual desire.

Deficiency and Excess

Deficiency (xu) and excess (shi) are two principles that help analyze and generalize the opposing forces between the body's resistance and pathogenic factors during the course of a disease. Basically, deficient (xu) indicate conditions caused by weakness and insufficiency of the body's resistance. Excess (shi) refer to conditions induced by an overabundance of pathogens.

Syndromes of Deficient (Xu) Type

This refers to conditions that are dominated by weakness of the body's disease preventing forces rather than by abundance of pathogenic factors. Owing to various disease preventing factors inside the body, patterns of deficiency (xu) can be further classified into such as qi deficiency, blood deficiency, yang deficiency, yin deficiency, body fluid deficiency, bone marrow depletion, nutrient stage deficiency and protective qi deficiency. Each of them has particular clinical features, some common signs of deficient syndromes are fatigue, low-spiritedness, pale or sallow complexion, palpitation, breath shortness, cold limbs, sweating, diarrhea, loose bowels, urinary frequency or incontinence. The tongue is pale, and the pulse is thready and weak. Deficient syndromes usually occur in those with constitutional defects, have chronic and ongoing diseases, or are in a depleted physical state.

Syndromes of Excess (Shi) Type

This refers to conditions that are dominated by abundance of pathogenic factors, the body's resistance has not yet weakened, resulting in hyperactive, precipitating struggles between the two forces. Besides exogenous pathogen invasions, excess syndromes can also be caused by internal damage such as qi stagnation, blood stasis, phlegm obstruction or stagnancy of fluid flow. Patients with an excess syndrome can develop complex symptoms, some common signs are fever, distension pain that becomes worse when pressed, chest stuffiness, irritability, coarse breathing, excessive throat discharges, constipation, urinary difficulty, and even unconsciousness. The tongue coating is thick and greasy, and the pulse is excess and forceful. Excess syndromes usually occur in those with a strong physique, newly developed cases, sudden attacks, and fierce clinical manifestations.

In reality, conditions that mix deficient and excess types are not uncommon. Excess and deficient syndromes are not steady, they can be transformed into each other, and may even appear fake signs to cover the underlying condition. For example, those who suffer from stagnation of blood and qi belong to an excess syndrome; however, when most of the body's disease preventing forces depleted, the body can be shifted to a mixed condition.

TCM physicians do not use the deficiency and excess principles alone, they are closely linked with another category – the cold and heat types. Excess type and heat type are often combined, while deficient type is combined with cold type.

Table: Cold & heat in relation to deficiency (xu) & excess (shi).

	Clinical features	Causes
Cold-excess type	Acute onset, chills, cold limbs, excess sputum, asthmatic breathing or breath shortness, abdominal pain that becomes worse when pressed, and constipation. The pulse is deep or taut and tense; the tongue may appear green-blue or purple color, and its coating is white, greasy and thick.	Invasion by exogenous cold; over-eating food with cold energies.
Cold-deficient type	Gradual onset, chills, cold limbs, breath shortness, general weakness, abdominal pain that can be alleviated by pressed, loose bowels, and clear profuse urine. The pulse is weak, deep and slow; the tongue is pale, bulky and tender.	Internal damages or long term illness leads to yang-qi depletion, and a relative excess of yin has developed inside the body. These are also termed as yang deficient syndrome.
Heat-excess type	Acute onset, relative short duration, persistent or high fever, thirst, red face, fullness and distending pain in the abdomen that becomes worse when pressed, constipation, urinary difficulty or yellow urine. There may also be unconsciousness in serious cases. The backside is hotter than the palm side when touching the hand, a rapid and excess pulse, the tongue is red or deep red with yellow coating.	Heat or fire evil invasion; over-eating spicy food or food with hot energies; excessive yang qi inside the body.
Heat-deficient type	Gradual onset, relative long duration, fluctuant low-grade fever, night sweating, bone pain, dry mouth, skinny appearance, breath shortness and general weakness. When touching the hand, the palm side is warmer than the backside. The pulse is thready and rapid; the tongue is red with little coating, or the tongue body may be bulky and tender.	Internal damages or long term illness leads to depletion of yin fluid and a relative excess of yang qi has formed inside the body. These are also called "virtual fire production" or "yin vacuity internal heat."

SPLEEN QI DEFICIENCY

Spleen qi refers not only to the actual organ called the spleen but to the entire digestive system and aspects of the circulatory system. Ordinarily, when the spleen qi is flowing properly, the digestive system also functions properly. Blood and all the fluids of the digestive system move smoothly, and there are no backups or sagging of the organs.

When the qi is blocked as a result of dampness, however, a number of symptoms can develop. Many of these symptoms relate to appetite and weight; others to fatigue and pale skin.

Western diagnoses associated with spleen qi deficiency include ulcers, gastritis, chronic fatigue, AIDS, chronic indigestion, and hepatitis. Note that these disorders must be medically diagnosed and treated as some of these conditions can be life-threatening.

Causes

According to Chinese Traditional Medicine, the spleen prefers a dry environment. Thus, dampness can cause issues with the spleen qi. For example, living in a damp climate or eating cold or raw foods can cause spleen dampness.

Symptoms

- Weakness, lethargy,
- Pale, bright face,
- Shallow breathing,
- Low, soft voice,
- Little desire to speak,
- Poor appetite,
- Prolonged headache,
- Fatigue,
- Loose stools,
- Lethargy,
- Dizziness,
- Tired eyes,
- Dislike cold greasy foods,

- Headache after exertion,
- Symptoms are worse in the morning,
- Abdominal discomfort which feels better when pressure is applied,
- Indigestion,
- Bloating and gas,
- Weak limbs.

Tongue Appearance

Pale or normal tongue. May have swollen sides.

Pulse

Weak pulse.

Related Conditions

- Gastric or duodenal ulcer,
- Dyspepsia,
- Hepatitis,
- Anemia.

Herbs that may Help

These are just some of the herbs that are believed to help spleen qi deficiency:

- Codonopsis,
- Ginseng (part of the traditional tonic called Four Gentlemen decoction),
- Astragalus,
- Jujube Dates.

Foods to Strengthen the Spleen

- Beef,
- Root vegetables,
- Warm foods,
- Soups,
- Warming spices, such as black pepper, ginger, cumin.

Treatments for Qi Deficiency

TCM places great importance on treating the body as a whole rather than merely managing symptoms. Where western medicine might treat tiredness with stimulants, such as coffee, TCM concerns itself with addressing the issues causing the fatigue in the first place.

There is little quality scientific research to support topics such as qi and qi deficiency, and most of the evidence for treating qi deficiency is anecdotal.

That said, many people may find relief from symptoms by making some changes in their diet and lifestyle to support their qi balance or using alternative therapies, such as acupuncture.

Focus on Rest

People with qi deficiency may work too hard, are always on the go, and never have downtime. To help balance the qi in the body, many TCM practitioners recommend a heavy focus on rest.

This can include:

- Taking breaks throughout the day.
- Making time to take a nap.
- Doing relaxing activities, such as yoga, tai chi, or qigong.

Improve Sleep Patterns

People with a qi deficiency may have a tendency towards stress and may benefit from improving their sleep patterns. A study published in Experimental Neurobiology reports that excessive stress is bad for both the body and the brain. Stress may activate the brain at night, making sound sleep difficult.

Reducing stress levels may help a person sleep better and have more energy or qi throughout the day. Try to find a set time to go to sleep and wake up each day, and aim to get at least 7 to 9 hours of sleep each night.

Best Foods for a Qi Deficiency

TCM suggests that a qi deficiency might be influenced by the spleen, which carries qi to other parts of the body. This is why a qi deficiency might occur in any area of the body.

To balance qi, TCM practitioners recommend eating foods that are good for the spleen.

Foods to Eat

A healthful diet for a balanced qi includes:

- Fermented foods for digestive health, including sauerkraut, kimchi, and kefir.

- Healthful, energizing fats, such as olive oil, salmon, coconut oil, and avocados.
- A wide variety of lightly cooked fruits, vegetables, and nuts.
- Adaptogenic herbs, such as ginseng, should be taken under the guidance of a healthcare practitioner or trusted TCM practitioner.

Foods that are good for spleen qi include yang tonic foods and qi-circulating foods. According to TCM, these foods might warm the spleen and increase energy flow to the body.

Foods to eat for spleen qi include:

- Lentils,
- Quinoa,
- Oats,
- Malted grain beverages,
- Root vegetables including sweet potato and taro,
- Pumpkin and other squash,
- Miso soup,
- Orange peels,
- Mustard leaf.

Foods to Avoid

Foods to avoid for spleen qi include:

- Refined sugar,
- Refined grains,
- Fried or salty foods,
- Iced or refrigerated foods or drinks,
- Dairy products,
- Citrus fruits,
- Pork,
- Yeasty foods, such as beer or dough,
- Banana.

References

- Causes-of-disease-in-chinese-medicine: agelessherbs.com, Retrieved 3 August, 2020

- Emotions-in-traditional-chinese-medicine-88196: verywellmind.com, Retrieved 16 January, 2020
- Traditional-chinese-medicine-diagnosis, chinese, natural-medicine, wellness: howstuffworks.com, Retrieved 29 March, 2020
- Yinyang: acupuncturetoday.com, Retrieved 2 June, 2020
- Diagnosis-eightprinciples, exam, eng, shen-nong.com, Retrieved 10 July, 2020
- Inflammation: chinesemedicineworks.com, Retrieved 23 February, 2020
- Spleen-qi-deficiency-89977: verywellhealth.com, Retrieved 13 March, 2020

Chinese Therapies

CHAPTER 6

The Chinese therapies are used for improving sleep quality, balancing hormones, reducing side effects of chemotherapy and radiation, treating neuropathy, stress, arthritis, etc. Some of the most common therapies are cupping, Gua sha, Tui na, Qigong, and Chinese food therapy. This chapter closely examines these therapies of traditional Chinese medicine to provide an extensive understanding of the subject.

CUPPING

Cupping was established as an official therapeutic practice in the 1950s across hospitals in China after research conducted by Chinese and former Soviet Union acupuncturists confirmed cupping's effectiveness. Prior to the 1950s, cupping had also been practiced as an auxiliary method in traditional Chinese surgery. In recent years cupping has been growing in popularity, with celebrities like Gwyneth Paltrow, Jennifer Aniston, David Arquette, and athlete Michael Phelps drawing public attention to the traditional Chinese therapy technique.

Though news outlets were quick to criticize celebrities chasing the newest medical therapies and techniques, recent studies have shown cupping's effectiveness in reducing pain intensity and providing positive short-term benefits.

Cupping is the term applied to a technique that uses small glass cups or bamboo jars as suction devices that are placed on the ski to disperse and break up stagnation and congestion by drawing congested blood, energy or other humors to the surface. In dry cupping, the therapist will simply place the suction cups on the skin. In wet cupping, the practitioner will make a small incision on the skin and then apply the suction cup to draw out small amounts of blood.

There are several ways that a practitioner can create the suction in the cups. One method involves swabbing rubbing alcohol onto the bottom of the cup, then lighting it and putting the cup immediately against the skin. Suction can also be created by placing an inverted cup over a small flame, or by using an alcohol-soaked cotton pad over an insulating material (like leather) to protect the skin, then lighting the pad and placing an empty cup over the flame to extinguish it. Flames are never used near the skin and are not lit throughout the process of cupping, but rather are a means to create the heat that causes the suction within the small cups.

Once the suction has occurred, the cups can be gently moved across the skin (often referred to as "gliding cupping). Medical massage oils are sometimes applied to improve movement of the glass cups along the skin. The suction in the cups causes the skin and superficial muscle layer to be lightly drawn into the cup. Cupping is much like the inverse of massage – rather than applying pressure to muscles, it uses gentle pressure to pull them upward. For most patients, this is a particularly relaxing and relieving sensation. Once suctioned, the cups are generally left in place for about ten minutes while the patient relaxes. This is similar to the practice of Tui Na, a traditional Chinese medicine massage technique that targets acupuncture points as well as painful body parts, and is well known to provide relief through pressure.

The side effects of cupping are fairly mild. Bruising should be expected, but skin should return to looking normal within 10 days. Other potential side effects include mild discomfort, skin infection, or burns. However, a trained health professional will apply an antibiotic ointment and bandage to prevent an infection.

Philosophy behind Pain and Cupping

"Where there's stagnation, there will be pain. Remove the stagnation, and you remove the pain." The old Chinese medical maxim holds that pain results from the congestion, stagnation, and blockage of Qi, or vital energy, vital fluids, lymph, phlegm, and blood. If pain is the essence of disease, then suffering is a result of obstructed or irregular flow in the body. Chinese cupping is therefore a method of breaking up the blockage to restore the body's natural flow of energy.

Cupping Combined with Acupuncture

Generally, cupping is combined with acupuncture in one treatment, but it can also be used alone. The suction and negative pressure provided by cupping can loosen muscles, encourage blood flow, and sedate the nervous system (which makes it an excellent treatment for high blood pressure). Cupping is used to relieve back and neck pains, stiff muscles, anxiety, fatigue, migraines, rheumatism, and even cellulite. For weight loss and cellulite treatments, oil is first applied to the skin, and then the cups are moved up and down the surrounding area.

Like acupuncture, cupping follows the lines of the meridians. There are five meridian lines on the back, and these are where the cups are usually placed. Using these points, cupping can help to align and relax qi, as well as target more specific maladies. By targeting the meridian channels, cupping strives to 'open' these channels – the paths through which life energy flows freely throughout the body, through all tissues and organs, thus providing a smoother and more free-flowing qi (life force). Cupping is one of the best deep-tissue therapies available. It is thought to affect tissues up to four inches deep from the external skin. Toxins can be released, blockages can be cleared, and veins and arteries can be refreshed within these four inches of affected materials. Even hands, wrists, legs, and ankles can be 'cupped,' thus applying the healing to specific organs that correlate with these points.

Other Benefits of Chinese Cupping

This treatment is also valuable for the lungs, and can clear congestion from a common cold or help to control a person's asthma. In fact, respiratory conditions are one of the most common maladies that cupping is used to relieve.

Cupping's detoxifying effect on skin and circulatory system is also significant, with a visible improvement in skin color after three to five treatments. Cupping removes toxins and improves blood flow through the veins and arteries. Especially useful for athletes is cupping's potential to relieve muscle spasms.

Cupping also affects the digestive system. A few benefits include an improved metabolism, relief from constipation, a healthy appetite, and stronger digestion.

Effectiveness

Cupping is poorly supported by scientific evidence, with a 2014 review of recent evidence finding that "because of the unreasonable design and poor research quality, the clinical evidence of cupping therapy is very low." A 2011 review found that "the effectiveness of cupping is currently not well-documented for most conditions", and that systematic reviews showing efficacy for the treatment of pain "were based mostly on poor quality primary studies." The American Cancer Society notes that "available scientific evidence does not support claims that cupping has any health benefits" and also that the treatment carries a small risk of burns.

Simon Singh and Edzard Ernst write that no evidence exists of any beneficial effects of cupping for any medical condition. Critics of alternative medicine such as Harriet Hall and Mark Crislip have characterized cupping as "pseudoscience nonsense", "a celebrity fad", and "gibberish", and observed that there is no evidence that cupping works any better than a placebo. Pharmacologist David Colquhoun writes that cupping is "laughable and utterly implausible." Practicing surgeon David Gorski observes, "it's all risk for no benefit. It has no place in modern medicine, or at least shouldn't."

Safety

While ineffective, cupping is generally safe when applied by trained professionals on people who are otherwise healthy. Cupping may result in bruising, burns, pain, and/or skin infection, and is not recommended for people with health problems due to side effects. In 2016, the Cambodian Ministry of Health warned that cupping could be a health risk and particularly dangerous for people with high blood pressure or heart problems.

Research suggests that cupping is harmful, especially in people who are thin or obese: According to Jack Raso, cupping results in capillary expansion, excessive fluid accumulation in tissues, and the rupture of blood vessels.

Cupping therapy adverse events can be divided into local and systemic adverse events. The local adverse events were scar formation, burns, skin infection, panniculitis, abscess formation, pain at the cupping site, and systemic adverse events including: anemia, dizziness, vasovagal attack, insomnia, headaches, and nausea.

Fire cupping can sometimes result in minor to severe burns at the cupping site, and may lead to hospitalization and may even require skin grafting to repair the injury. Other burns can also occur due to carelessness with the flammable substances being used, such as spills and over application.

Some contraindications for cupping may include: pregnancy, swelling, dry or cracked skin, hypotension, open wounds, or thin blood.

Methods

While details vary between practitioners, societies, and cultures, the practice consists of drawing tissue into a cap placed on the targeted area by creating a partial vacuum – either by the heating and subsequent cooling of the air in the cup, or via a mechanical pump. The cup is usually left in place for somewhere between five and fifteen minutes.

Cupping therapy types can be classified using four distinct methods of categorisation. The first system of categorisation relates to "technical types" including: dry, wet, massage, and flash cupping therapy. The second categorisation relates to "the power of suction related types" including: light, medium, and strong cupping therapy. The third categorisation relates to "the method of suction related types" including: fire, manual suction, and electrical suction cupping therapy. The fourth categorisation relates to "materials inside cups" including: herbal products, water, ozone, moxa, needle, and magnetic cupping therapy.

Further categories of cupping were developed later. The fifth relates to area treated including: facial, abdominal, female, male, and orthopedic cupping therapy. The sixth relates to "other cupping types" that include sports and aquatic cupping.

Cups of Various Materials:

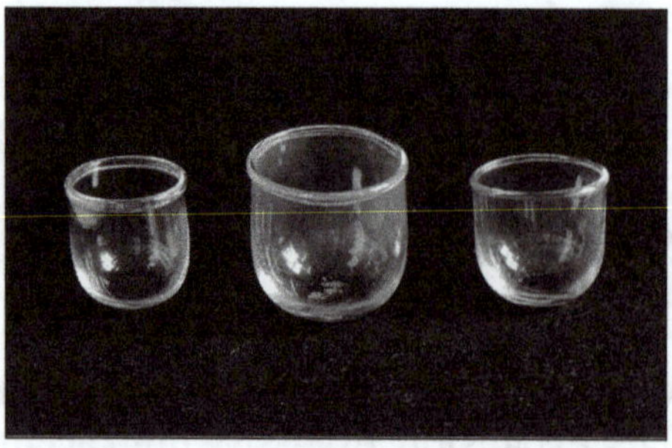

Glass.

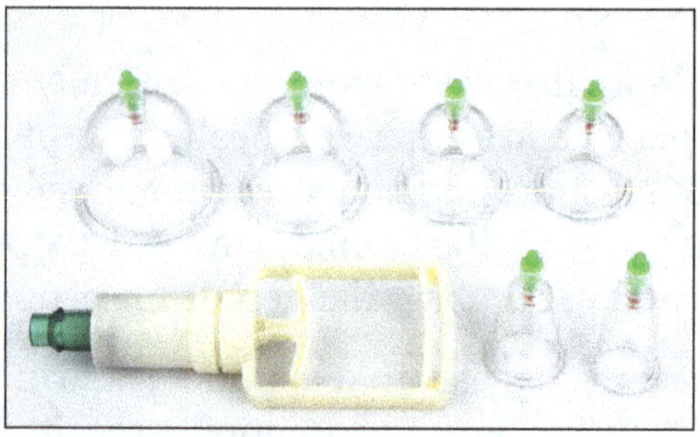

Plastic.

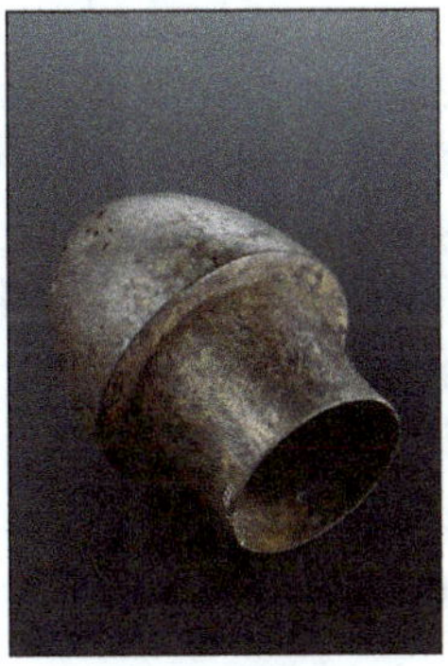

Bronze.

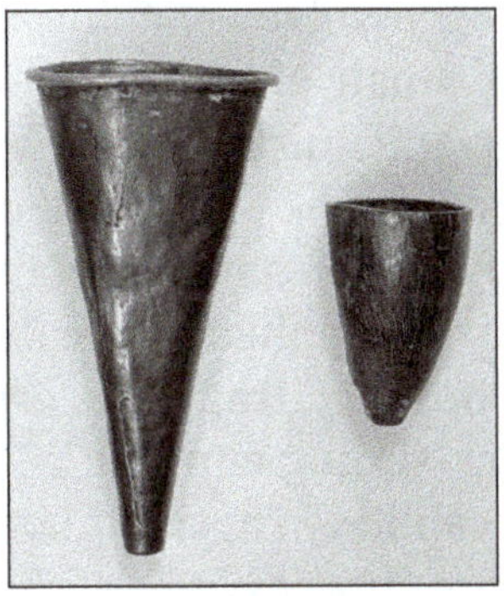

Horn/Copper.

Dry Cupping

The cupping procedure commonly involves creating a small area of low air pressure next to the skin. However, there are varieties in the tools used, the methods of creating the low pressure, and the procedures followed during the treatment.

The cups can be of various shapes including balls or bells, and may range in size from 1 to 3 inches (25 to 76 mm) across the opening. Plastic and glass are the most common materials used today, replacing the horn, pottery, bronze and bamboo cups used in earlier times. The low air pressure required may be created by heating the cup or the air inside it with an open flame or a bath in hot scented oils, then placing it against the skin. As the air inside the cup cools, it contracts and draws the skin slightly inside. More recently, vacuum is created with a mechanical suction pump acting through a valve located at the top of the cup. Rubber cups are also available that squeeze the air out and adapt to uneven or bony surfaces.

In practice, cups are normally used only on softer tissue that can form a good seal with the edge of the cup. They may be used singly or with many to cover a larger area. They may be used by themselves or placed over an acupuncture needle. Skin may be lubricated, allowing the cup to move across the skin slowly.

Fire Cupping

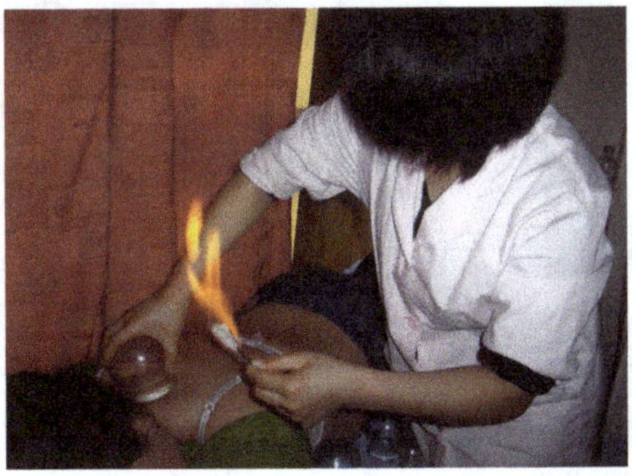

A person receiving fire cupping.

Fire cupping involves soaking a cotton ball in almost pure alcohol. The cotton is clamped by a pair of forceps and lit via match or lighter, and, in one motion, placed into the cup and quickly removed, while the cup is placed on the skin. The fire uses up all the oxygen in the cup which creates a negative pressure inside the cup. The cup is then quickly placed onto the body and the negative pressure "sucks" the skin up. Massage oil may be applied to create a better seal as well as allow the cups to glide over muscle groups (e.g. trapezius, erectors, latissimus dorsi, etc.) in an act called "gliding cupping" or "sliding cupping". Dark circles may appear where the cups were placed because of capillary rupture just under the skin. There are documented cases of burns caused by fire cupping.

Wet Cupping

Wet cupping is also known as Hijama or medicinal bleeding, where blood is drawn by local suction from a small skin incision.

Wet cupping, unlike dry cupping, requires a skin incision. The skin incision can be made either before or after cupping treatment. The cup is meant to suck out any impurities in the body which may include blood, toxins, fragmented blood cells, and tissue fluid.

The first reported usages are found in the Islamic hadith, sayings attributed to or describing the actions of the Islamic prophet Muhammad. Hadith from Muhammad al-Bukhari, Muslim ibn al-Hajjaj Nishapuri and Ahmad ibn Hanbal support its recommendation and use by Muhammad. As a result, wet cupping has remained a popular remedy practiced in many parts of the Muslim world.

In Finland, wet cupping has been done at least since the 15th century, and it is done traditionally in saunas. The cupping cups were made of cattle horns with a valve mechanism in it to create a partial vacuum by sucking the air out. Cupping is still practiced in Finland as part of relaxing and/or health regimens.

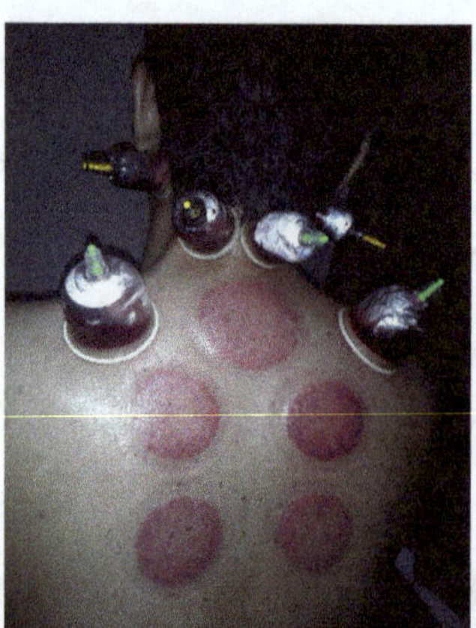

A person receiving wet cupping.

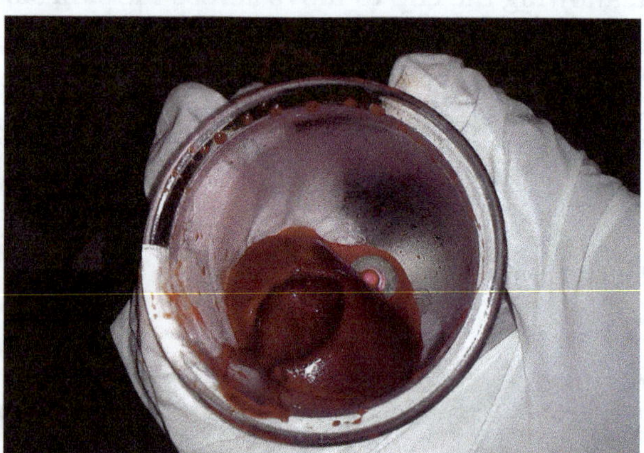

Blood drawn by wet cupping.

Traditional Chinese Medicine

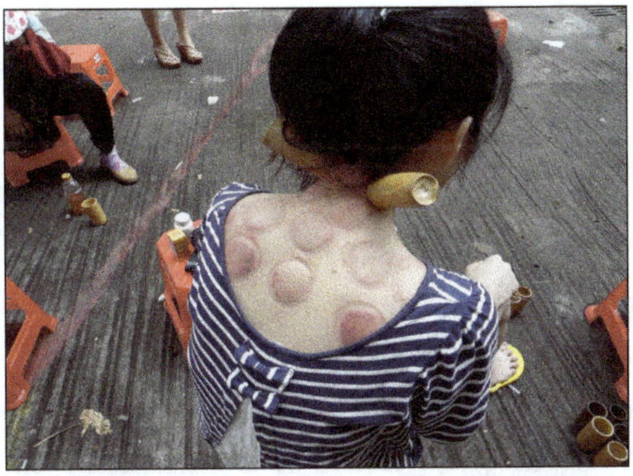

Woman receiving fire cupping at a roadside business in Haikou, Hainan, China.

According to traditional Chinese medicine (TCM), cupping is done to dispel stagnation (stagnant blood and lymph), thereby improving qi flow, in order to treat respiratory diseases such as the common cold, pneumonia and bronchitis. Cupping also is used on back, neck, shoulder and other musculoskeletal conditions. Its advocates claim it has other applications as well. Cupping is not advised, in TCM, over skin ulcers or to the abdominal or sacral regions of pregnant women

GUA SHA

Gua sha is a natural, alternative therapy that involves scraping your skin with a massage tool to improve your circulation. This ancient Chinese healing technique may offer a unique approach to better health, addressing issues like chronic pain.

In gua sha, a technician scrapes your skin with short or long strokes to stimulate microcirculation of the soft tissue, which increases blood flow. They make these strokes with a smooth-edged instrument known as a gua massage tool. The technician applies massage oil to your skin, and then uses the tool to repeatedly scrape your skin in a downward motion.

Gua sha is intended to address stagnant energy, called chi, in the body that practitioners believe may be responsible for inflammation. Inflammation is the underlying cause of several conditions associated with chronic pain. Rubbing the skin's surface is thought to help break up this energy, reduce inflammation, and promote healing.

Gua sha is generally performed on a person's back, buttocks, neck, arms, and legs. A gentle version of it is even used on the face as a facial technique. Your technician may apply mild pressure, and gradually increase intensity to determine how much force you can handle.

What are the Benefits of Gua Sha?

Gua sha may reduce inflammation, so it's often used to treat ailments that cause chronic pain, such as arthritis and fibromyalgia, as well as those that trigger muscle and joint pain.

Gua sha may also relieve symptoms of other conditions:

Hepatitis B

Hepatitis B is a viral infection that causes liver inflammation, liver damage, and liver scarring. Research suggests that gua sha may reduce chronic liver inflammation.

One case followed a man with high liver enzymes, an indicator of liver inflammation. He was given gua sha, and after 48 hours of treatment he experienced a decline in liver enzymes. This leads researchers to believe that gua sha has the ability to improve liver inflammation, thus decreasing the likelihood of liver damage. More research is underway.

Migraine Headaches

If your migraine headaches don't respond to over-the-counter medications, gua sha may help. In one, a 72-year-old woman living with chronic headaches received gua sha over a 14-day period. Her migraines improved during this time, suggesting that this ancient healing technique may be an effective remedy for headaches. More research is needed.

Breast Engorgement

Breast engorgement is a condition experienced by many breastfeeding women. This is when the breasts overfill with milk. It usually occurs in the first weeks of breastfeeding or if the mother is away from the infant for any reason. Breasts become swollen and painful, making it difficult for babies to latch. This is usually a temporary condition.

In one, women were given gua sha from the second day after giving birth up until leaving the hospital. The hospital followed up with these women in the weeks after giving birth and found that many had fewer reports of engorgement, breast fullness, and discomfort. This made it easier for them to breastfeed.

Neck Pain

Gua sha technique may also prove effective for remedying chronic neck pain. To determine the effectiveness of this therapy, 48 study participantsTrusted Source were split into two groups. One group was given gua sha and the other used a thermal heating pad to treat neck pain. After one week, participants who received gua sha reported less pain compared to the group that didn't receive gua sha.

Tourette Syndrome

Tourette syndrome involves involuntary movements such as facial tics, throat clearing, and vocal outbursts. According to a single case, gua sha combined with other therapies may have helped to reduce symptoms of Tourette syndrome in the study participant.

The study involved a 33-year-old male who had Tourette syndrome since the age of 9. He received acupuncture, herbs, gua sha, and modified his lifestyle. After 35 once-a-week treatments, his symptoms improved by 70 percent. Even though this man had positive results, further research is needed.

Perimenopausal Syndrome

Perimenopause occurs as women move closer to menopause. Symptoms include:

- Insomnia.
- Irregular periods.
- Anxiety.
- Fatigue.
- Hot flashes.

One, however, found that gua sha may reduce symptoms of perimenopause in some women.

The study examined 80 women with perimenopausal symptoms. The intervention group received 15 minute gua sha treatments once a week in conjunction with conventional therapy for eight weeks. The control group only received conventional therapy.

Upon completion of the study, the intervention group reported greater reduction of symptoms such as insomnia, anxiety, fatigue, headaches, and hot flashes compared to the control group. Researchers believe gua sha therapy might be a safe, effective remedy for this syndrome.

Does Gua Sha have Side Effects?

As a natural healing remedy, gua sha is safe. It's not supposed to be painful, but the procedure may change the appearance of your skin. Because it involves rubbing or scraping skin with a massage tool, tiny blood vessels known as capillaries near the surface of your skin can burst. This can result in skin bruising and minor bleeding. Bruising usually disappears within a couple of days.

Some people also experience temporary indentation of their skin after a gua sha treatment.

If any bleeding occurs, there's also the risk of transferring bloodborne illnesses with gua sha therapy, so it's important for technicians to disinfect their tools after each person.

Avoid this technique if you've had any surgery in the last six weeks.

People who are taking blood thinners or have clotting disorders aren't good candidates for gua sha.

CHINESE FOOD THERAPY AND MEDICAL DIET

Food therapy of traditional Chinese medicine aims to maintain balanced nutrition through diet. Medical diet therapy, however, is to achieve the balance of Yin and Yang through the combination of nutrition and medicine. Either "food therapy" or "medical diet therapy" aims to keep health, prevent disease, remove illness and slow aging. In recent years, both food therapy and medical diet therapy have been increasingly applied in clinical nutrition therapy.

Food therapy of traditional medicine aims to maintain balanced nutrition through diet. Medical diet therapy, however, is to achieve the balance of Yin and Yang through the combination of nutrition and medicine. There are both connections and distinctions between them. On the basis of traditional food therapy, medical diet therapy coordinates with drugs and adopts traditional culinary skills and modern processing methods to produce food, which is not only with terrific color, aroma, taste and shape but also health-keeping, disease-resisting and healing as well as longevity-promoting. It treats through eating, that is, medicine can be used as food and food can be combined with medicine. In this way, medicine functions by means of food and food reinforces the effects of medicine. To this extent, medicine and food supplement and bring out the best in each other through combination. Either "food therapy" or "medical diet therapy" aims to keep health, prevent disease, remove illness and slow aging.

Long before, plenty of monographs appeared in masterpieces of Traditional Chinese Medicine, like Canon of Yellow Emperor, Shennong's Classic of Materia Medica, Invaluable Prescriptions for Ready Reference, Principles of Correct Diet, discussing how diet plays a role in human's physiology, pathology, health maintenance and disease treatment. For example, in Plain Questions: On Soup and Mash, it is recorded that grains were boiled into soup, as nourishment to the five internal organs (heart, liver, spleen, lung and kidney) in ancient times. After boiling for some time, grains were fermented and turned into mash, which can be used as treatment to the above five internal organs.

With the rapid growth of people's living standard and working pace, more and more attention and recognition are paid to the adjuvant therapeutic effects of food therapy and medical diet therapy, that is, health maintenance and disease avoidance. In recent years, both food therapy and medical diet therapy have been increasingly applied in clinical nutrition therapy. In terms of traditional Chinese food therapy and medical diet therapy, their clinical applications principles are summarized as follows.

Food Therapy—To Fully Cure Disease, Eat Grains, Meat, fruit and Vegetables

Written more than 2000 years ago, Plain Questions: On Laws and Times of Organs had already pointed out that grains to nourish, fruit to assist, livestock to benefit, vegetables to supplement, take them in proper proportion to supply energy. The key point is to keep a balanced diet. Besides, it has suggested that when one's illness is already under control, it could be removed gradually by eating grains, meat, fruit and vegetables. There is no more need to take too much medicine, which might cause extreme side effects to our health. The claimed "grains to nourish" refers to using millet, sorghum, beans, wheat, rice and other cereals and beans as staple food for maintaining one's life. "Fruit to assist" means that Li, apricot, chestnut, peach and other fruits and nuts are essential food aid to balanced diet. "Livestock to benefit" emphasizes that cattle, dogs, sheep, pigs, chicken and other livestock are beneficial to human body along with making up the deficiency of nutrition that grains can't provide. They serve as the main complementary food in the balanced diet recipe. "Vegetables to supplement" indicates that vegetables like kwai, leek, allium, scallion, shallot etc. can supplement various essential nutrients.

In other words, grains, meat, vegetables and fruit should be used in proper proportions so as to maintain the normal function of human body. Moreover, following a diet is very necessary and it is not advisable to either starve or overeat. Starvation will cause insufficiency of vital energy and blood and decline of immunity, resulting in diseases, such as malnutrition, anemia. According to Plain Questions: On Arthralgia, intestines and stomach would be impaired by overeating, along with symptoms like abdominal fullness and distention, anorexia, excessive gastric acid and vomiting and diarrhea. Therefore, Traditional Chinese Medicine emphasizes that it is necessary for people to keep a regular diet habit and arrange balanced diet according to one's age, gender and constitution. This viewpoint is exactly consistent with the balanced diet proposed by experts of modern nutriology.

Traditional Medicine holds that food has various properties, including warm, hot, cold, cool. Among them, warm and hot share the same property, while cold and cool are of the same nature. Warm and hot food can warm the spleen and stomach for dispelling coldness, invigorate the spleen and reinforce the stomach, and reinforce the kidney-yang, which are suitable for those who are in deficiency of Yang with hyperactivity of Yin and cold constitution, with symptoms appearing like cold limbs and waist, chills, thin sloppy stool and frequent nocturia. Warm food mainly includes glutinous rice, oats, red dates, arillus longan, pine nut, garlic, chives, onion, coffee, black tea and chicken, etc. Hot food basically includes pepper, cinnamon, mutton, venison, etc. Both cold and cool food possess positive effects, for instance, clearing heat and purging fire, detoxifying and laxative, expelling damp and dryness, which are beneficial to those in deficiency of Yin and with hyperactivity of Yang and hot constitution, with symptoms like repeated sore mouth and tongue, dry mouth and tongue, dysphoria with feverish sensation in chest, palms and soles, and dry stool, etc. Cool food mainly involves millet, mung bean, pear, mango, loquat, lily, tomato, eggplant, tofu, lotus root, wax gourd, chrysanthemum, milk, and rabbit, etc. Cold food includes watermelon, bitter gourd, kelp, nori, water spinach, honeysuckle and aloe, etc. In addition, there is some mild food, neither cold nor hot and good to eat all year round, for instance, rice, corn, sesame, soybean, cowpea, pea, apple, pineapple, grape, peanut, radish, Chinese yam, mushroom, pork, lycium barbarum, etc.

Food does not only possess the above four properties, that is, warm, hot, cold and cool, but also carry with five flavors, viz., spicy, sweet, sour, bitter, salty. According to Plain Questions: On Five Flavors, talking about distributions of five flavors, sour food was said to be absorbed by the liver, spicy by the lungs, bitter by the heart, salty by the kidney, sweet by the spleen. That is to say, each flavor plays a different role in different organs respectively. Disordered diet or being partially addicted to a particular food will do harm to the above mentioned five organs. In Plain Questions: On Vigor and Nature, it's been mentioned that on the one hand, Yin originates from five flavors, however, on the other hand, organs where Yin is stored could also be impaired by overuse of five flavors. If it is too sour, the liver-qi would increase and the spleen-qi will decrease. If too salty, it could lead to bone damage, impotent muscle and depressed heart-qi; if too sweet, the heart-qi would rise up, causing asthma, darkened skin and imbalance of the kidney-qi; if too bitter, it could cause dryness of the spleen-qi, bloating of stomach; if too spicy, tendons and vessels would become flabby and vigor would be undermined. That is to say, physiological condition and pathological mechanism of the five internal organs are inseparable from the five flavors of food. He pointed out that being a doctor, the first thing is to know clearly the source of the disease, what the symptom is and treat with food therapy. If food therapy fails, then prescribe medicine. This concept indicates that food therapy should be used before medication therapy, which theoretically supports the view, "dietetic nourishment should be used in preference to medical invigoration."

Medical Therapy—Harmonize Yin-Yang to Balance

Traditional Chinese Medicine believes that a state of health signifies the balance of Yin-Yang, while a condition of pathological state implies imbalance of Yin-Yang. As it is said in Plain Questions: On Regulation of Menstruation, if Yin and Yang have been in a balance, it will be shown in his physique; if the nine pulse taking sites functions as one, he shall be considered to be healthy. On the contrary, "excessive Yin causes Yang disease, vice versa, excessive Yang causes Yin disease. Predominance of Yang brings about heat syndrome, vice versa, predominance of Yin brings about cold syndrome", stated in Plain Questions: On Yin-Yang Regulations. Hence, "the basis of proper treatment needs to figure out the status of Yin-Yang. Then regulate it into balance", recorded in Plain Questions: True Essence. Traditional Chinese Medical diet therapy is exactly conceived under the guidance of holistic theory, whose core is Yin-Yang balance. By means of making up deficiency of one side and controlling excessiveness of the other side, Traditional Chinese medical diet therapy aims to bring Yin-Yang back to a relatively balanced state.

The so-called "controlling excessiveness" mainly targets at constitutions or symptoms with excessive Yin. For heat syndrome caused by excessive Yang heat, medical diet therapy suggests to "expelling heat with cold herbs". For example, choose reed rhizome, lotus leaf, mung bean and other medicine of cold nature to make porridge or soup so as to clear away heat (Yang). For cold syndrome caused by excessive Yin cold, medical diet therapy suggests to "treat cold with hot herbs". For example, add cinnamon, dry ginger, fennel to make porridge or soup so as to dispel cold (Yin). Yet the alleged "making up deficiency" is mainly applied for constitutions or symptoms with deficient Yin or Yang. When dealing with deficient heat syndrome resulting from deficient Yin, medical diet therapy recommends to "use cold-nature herbs to restrain Yang". For example, add radix asparagus, radix ophiopogonis, lily, radix polygonati officinalis, etc. into cooking to nourish Yin and inhibit Yang. When dealing with deficient cold syndrome resulting from deficient Yang, medical diet therapy advises to "boost the source of heat to eliminate Yin". For example, stew mutton meat with antler gelatin, radix aconiti lateralis preparata, nourishing Yang to restrain Yin. Just as in this way, food therapy should adopt according to conditions of Yin-Yang and diet should be properly arranged to maintain the balance between Yin and Yang.

Treatment in Accordance with Three Categories of Etiologic Factors

The essence of three categories of etiologic factors refers to treat individually-oriented, climate-oriented and locality-oriented. It means that to achieve the expected therapeutic effects, what to eat should be tailored to the needs of corresponding constitution, age, gender, region and other situations.

Climate-oriented

Just as the four seasons are graded as cold, hot, warm and cool, the properties of food and medicine also vary from one to another, including refreshing, light, pungent and mild tonic. Accordingly, either food therapy or medical diet therapy should be adjusted in different seasons so as to comply with the natural laws of climate changes. Human's activities should be in accordance with the following rule: "sow in spring; grow in summer; harvest in autumn; store in winter". As per recommendations in Principles of Correct Diet, written by imperial physician Hu Sihui of Yuan Dynasty, "warm in spring, suitable for eating wheat to cool; hot in summer, suitable for eating mung beans to chill; dry in autumn, suitable for eating sesame to nourish dryness; cold in winter, suitable for eating broomcorn millet to dispel cold.

Spring is a good time to nourish growth and development qi. So it's better to eat those can sooth the liver in order to keep liver and other organs functioning normally. For instance, Chinese chives taste pungent but warm in nature. Its pungent taste assists to disperse liver qi and its warm nature is helpful to warm Yang and tonify the weak. This also conforms to the theory, viz., "nourish Yang in spring and summer". Meanwhile, people ought to cut down their intake of sour food and increase that of sweet food. It's better to tonify the spleen with sweet food, like Chinese yam, lycium barbarum, sweet potato, etc.

In summer, the climate is hot. So it is advisable to treat heat syndrome with cold, using food which can clear heat, nourish Yin and promote the production of body fluid, such as watermelon, fresh lotus root, mung bean and cucumber, etc. They had better reduce bitter food and increase pungent food to nourish the lungs. The long summer stands between summer and autumn, both hot and damp. The dampness in the air reaches the peak during this period. Thus, it's better to choose ingredients that can invigorate the spleen and eliminate dampness, for example, Poria cocos, coix seed, wax gourd, semen lablab album, lotus seed, etc.

When autumn comes, everything begins to converge as the climate turns cool and dry. It's time to nourish lungs with moistening food, such as, pear, lily, loquat, etc. In autumn, people ought to eat less pungent food but intake more sour food in order to drop off lung qi and benefit liver qi. Therefore during autumn, ginger, garlic, scallion with pungency should be lessened while sour food like dark plum, hawthorn, grape, should be encouraged.

In winter, the air is mainly filled with coldness. Thus, it's time to "expel cold with heat", suitable for eating warm and hot food, like mutton, chicken, etc.

Locality-oriented

"Locality-oriented" refers to using different food therapy or medical diet therapy according to different regions. Climate, natural environment and living habit of different regions have different influence on human body's physiological activity and pathological changes. In cold and dry highland, where is often occupied with coldness and dryness, it's better to eat pungent and nourishing food or crude medicine. For example, fresh ginger, allium fistulosum, perilla leaf, cassia, mutton, etc. are favorable. However, in those hot and rainy, low and humid places, where is bathed in high humidity and heat, it's better to choose heat-clearing and damp-expelling food or crude medicine. For example, coix seed, cardamom fruit, ageratum, mint, villious amomum, etc.

Individual-oriented

Treatment in accordance with patient's individuality means to nurse his or her body by selecting those food or medicine based on individual constitution, age, gender and lifestyle. For instance, in terms of constitution, Yang-deficient people need to recuperate with warm food, such as mutton porridge. Yin-deficient people need to revitalize with nourishing food, such as tremella soup, radix ophiopogonis porridge. Qi-deficient people should be supplied with qi. It's necessary to try ginseng porridge, astragalus soup. Blood-deficient people had better to enrich the blood. Drinking soup that made from Chinese angelica and mutton would be a good choice. As for phlegmatic hygrosis patients, who are in need of dispelling phlegm, they should try porridge made from Pinellia ternate and Chinese yam.

In respect of age, children are vigorous, "Yang often excesses and Yin is often in deficiency". So do not administer invigorators to them. Their illnesses mostly result from excessive heat. In this case, food therapy or medical diet therapy should focus on clearing heat and diminishing fire. As for the aged, the functions of their viscera weaken gradually, causing insufficiency of qi and blood. They get sick mostly due to their deficiency of essential nutrients. The proper solution is to restore with invigorators.

As another example, men and women appear to be different physiologically and pathologically because of different gender. Women are confronted with menstruation, leucorrhea, pregnancy and parturition, which should be taken into consideration when adopting food therapy or medical diet therapy. For example, during their menstrual period and gestation period, food therapy generally focuses on supplementing Yin and blood. Egg, E Jiao (Colla Corii Asini) would be desirable in this case. Meanwhile, avoid food or medicine which is too hot, too cold, blood activating or purgative.

TUI NA

Tuina or tui-na massage originated in ancient China and is believed to be the oldest system of bodywork. It's one of the four main branches of traditional Chinese medicine, along with acupuncture, qi gong, and Chinese herbal medicine.

It's based on the theory that imbalances of qi, which is the body's vital life force or energy, can cause blockages or imbalances that lead to symptoms such as pain and illness.

Tuina massage stimulates the flow of qi to promote balance and harmony within the body using many of the same principles of acupuncture.

It's similar to acupuncture in the way it targets specific acupoints, but practitioners use fingers instead of needles to apply pressure to stimulate these points. Tuina massage is often used in combination with acupuncture.

How it Works?

The philosophy and principles of tuina massage are based on traditional Chinese medicine, which focuses on emotional and physical components of a person's well-being, as well as aspects such as climate, relationships, and diet.

The underlying philosophy of tuina massage is that true health is achieved when one has found harmony and balance inside the self and their environment.

The goal of tuina massage is to create harmony in the yin and yang of the body by getting rid of blockages and disturbances that manifest as illness, disease, and emotional issues.

Similar to acupuncture, tuina massage uses the same energetic meridians and acupoints to balance the qi and blood in your body, leading to better health. Qi that's flowing incorrectly can cause blockages, such as poor blood circulation in the affected area.

The main therapeutic goal of tuina massage is to remove the energetic blocks that are causing qi stagnation.

Technique

During a session, practitioners use oscillating and pressure techniques that differ in force and speed. Tuina massage can be done as a stronger deep-tissue massage or a more gentle, energetic treatment.

Some techniques are more yin, which is more gentle, passive, and meditative. The yang approach is more active, dynamic, and physical, creating more intense sensations by stimulating deep blockages and knots.

The practitioner massages the muscles and tendons and uses manipulation techniques to realign the body. Passive joint movements are used to restore function to muscles and joints.

Depending on your practitioner as well as your specific needs, various techniques will be used in a session. To enhance the effects of the treatment, herbal poultices or compresses, lotions, and salves are used.

Tuina massage uses massage techniques such as acupressure, myofascial release, and reflexology. Sometimes, techniques that are common to osteopathy and chiropractic, such as stretching and joint mobilizations, are also used.

There are eight basic techniques used in tuina massage:

- Palpating (mo).
- Rejoining (jie).
- Opposing (duan).
- Lifting (ti).
- Pressing (an).
- Kneading (mo).
- Pushing (tui).

- Holding (na).

Other techniques include:

- Rolling: This is used for injuries such as sprains and strains.
- One-finger technique: This is one-finger stimulation of acupressure points.
- Nei gung: This is a full-body manipulation technique.

What does it Treat?

Tuina massage can be used to treat specific health concerns or areas in the body. Since tuina massage is considered to be an alternative treatment, it's essential that you talk to your doctor before using it to treat any medical condition.

Tuina massage can be used to treat pain and illness, or to maintain good health. The technique is effective in reducing stress, encouraging relaxation, and deepening sleep. It's often used for conditions and injuries related to the musculoskeletal and nervous systems.

Here are some conditions tuina massage can treat:

- Neck and back pain.
- Musculoskeletal disorders.
- Premenstrual syndrome.
- Fatigue and insomnia.
- Carpal tunnel.
- Headaches.
- Arthritis.
- Osteoporosis.
- Stress.
- Digestive conditions.
- Respiratory conditions.

Benefits

While some of the research is preliminary and ongoing, there's plenty of evidence to back the effectiveness of tuina massage in treating health conditions. Let's see what some of the studies say about the benefits.

Boosts Blood Circulation

One of the main intentions of tuina massage is to boost blood circulation by stimulating the body's energy flow.

Yi Zhi chan tuina manipulation on BL 56 acupoint is effective in improving circulation. In this study, manipulation using medium force for 10 minutes was found to be more effective than treatments using light or heavy force for shorter amounts of time.

Larger studies are needed to expand on these findings.

Reduces Neck Pain

Tuina massage relieves neck pain and the accompanying tension, tightness, and irritation.

tuina massage is a cost-effective option for reducing pain in people with chronic neck pain. People who received six tuina treatments within three weeks reduced the intensity of their neck pain more than people who had no treatment.

Further research that compares tuina to other treatments is necessary, though.

Relieves Low Back Pain

Tuina massage can relieve lower back pain, especially when treatment is paired with core exercises.

Tuina massage was more effective when combined with core stability exercises in people with low back pain.

People who did tuina massage alone had higher rates of back pain at follow-up compared to people who incorporated core exercises to their treatment.

Treats Depression

Focusing on whole-body healing is essential for people with depression, since the causes can be both physical and emotional.

Studies concluded that tuina massage has a therapeutic effect on depression. It was shown to be significantly more effective in reducing depression than conventional treatments.

More high-quality studies are needed to confirm and expand on these findings.

Promotes Healthy Lactation

Tuina massage is used to encourage postpartum lactation.

The results showed that tuina massage on breasts increased the quantity of lactation compared to women who received only conventional treatment.

Though no significant difference was found between the groups in terms of delaying the decrease of prolactin levels, researchers believe tuina massage could have a positive effect in this area. It could help new mothers produce greater quantities of milk more quickly.

Treats Osteoarthritis

The therapeutic benefits of tuina massage extend to alleviating symptoms of osteoarthritis.

Trusted Source, it improves muscular tension of the flexor and extensor muscles in people with knee osteoarthritis. The treatment used gun, an, na, and ca maneuvers. The patients received treatments three times per week over the course of nine months.

Patients saw improvement in pain, stiffness, and function.

Eases Carpal Tunnel Syndrome

According to tuina massage can relieve symptoms from carpal tunnel syndrome.

People with carpal tunnel syndrome who received warm-needling acupuncture in addition to tuina massage showed significantly more improvements than people who were treated using hormone block therapy and medication.

Treats Musculoskeletal Disorders

Tuina massage is often used to improve function and reduce pain affecting the joints, bones, and muscles.

The effectiveness of tuina massage in treating musculoskeletal disorders. The technique was shown to be effective in relieving pain, especially compared to traction, medication, and physical therapies.

Evidence to support better function wasn't as strong as pain reduction. Further research is needed to expand on these findings.

Benefits Foot Issues from Diabetes

Tuina massage can be beneficial for people with diabetes who have foot issues.

Tuina massage combined with a Chinese medicine foot bath was therapeutically beneficial for people with early-stage diabetic foot.

People who received tuina massage and a foot bath in addition to conventional medicine showed significant improvements compared to people who received only conventional medicine.

Improves Quality of Life in Cancer Patients

Tuina massage is a viable option for people with cancer who want to manage symptoms related to the disease and its conventional treatment.

The effect of tuina massage on improving symptoms and quality of life for people with cancer. The meta-analysis also looked at the effects of:

- Acupuncture.
- Tai chi.
- Qi gong.
- Traditional Chinese medicine five-element music therapy.

When combined with acupuncture, tuina massage was effective in improving quality of life in people with terminal cancer. Tuina massage was also shown to be effective in relieving stomach discomfort.

Though tuina massage shows promise as a therapy to treat people with cancer, more in-depth research is needed, as many of the studies had limitations.

Side Effects

Tuina massage is a safe treatment and is generally well-tolerated. However, remember that it's not a gentle or relaxing massage, and you may feel some discomfort during or after a session. Slight bruising is possible.

It's not recommended for people who have fractures or are prone to fractures, vein inflammation, or any type of open wound. It's also not recommended for people with previous chronic back issues, such as ankylosing spondylitis.

QIGONG

Qigong is a holistic system of coordinated body-posture and movement, breathing, and meditation used for the purposes of health, spirituality, and martial-arts training. With roots in Chinese medicine, philosophy, and martial arts, qigong is traditionally viewed as a practice to cultivate and balance qi (pronounced approximately as "chi"), translated as "life energy".

Qigong practice typically involves moving meditation, coordinating slow-flowing movement, deep rhythmic breathing, and a calm meditative state of mind. People practise qigong throughout China and worldwide for recreation, exercise, relaxation, preventive medicine, self-healing, alternative medicine, meditation, self-cultivation, and training for martial arts.

Researchers have examined qigong in connection with a wide range of medical conditions (including hypertension, pain, and cancer) and with respect to quality of life. Most research concerning postulated health benefits of qigong has been of poor quality, such that it would be unwise to draw firm conclusions at this stage.

Qigong (Pinyin), ch'i kung (Wade-Giles), and chi gung (Yale) are English words for two Chinese characters: qì and gōng

Qi (or chi) is often translated as life energy, referring to energy circulating through the body; though a more general definition is universal energy, including heat, light, and electromagnetic energy; and definitions often involve breath, air, gas, or the relationship between matter, energy, and spirit. Qi is the central underlying principle in traditional Chinese medicine and martial arts. Gong (or kung) is often translated as cultivation or work, and definitions include practice, skill, mastery, merit, achievement, service, result, or accomplishment, and is often used to mean gongfu (kung fu) in the traditional sense of achievement through great effort. The two words are combined to describe systems to cultivate and balance life energy, especially for health.

The term qigong as currently used was promoted in the late 1940s through the 1950s to refer to a broad range of Chinese self-cultivation exercises, and to emphasize health and scientific approaches, while de-emphasizing spiritual practices, mysticism, and elite lineages.

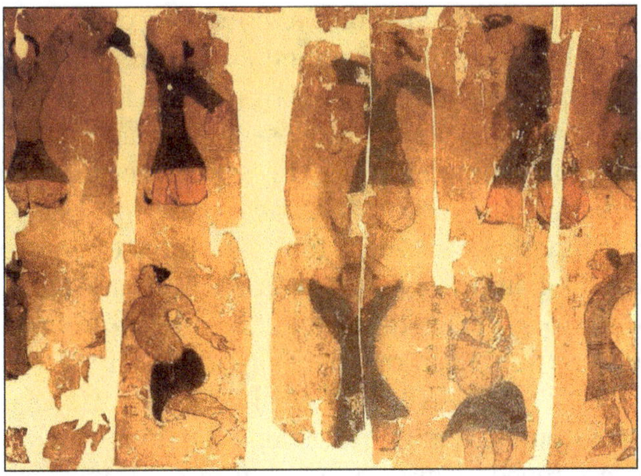

The physical exercise chart; a painting on silk depicting the practice of Qigong Taiji; unearthed in 1973 in Hunan Province, China.

With roots in ancient Chinese culture dating back more than 4,000 years, a wide variety of qigong forms have developed within different segments of Chinese society: in traditional Chinese medicine for preventive and curative functions; in Confucianism to promote longevity and improve moral character; in Daoism and Buddhism as part of meditative practice; and in Chinese martial arts to enhance fighting abilities. Contemporary qigong blends diverse and sometimes disparate traditions, in particular the Daoist meditative practice of "internal alchemy", the ancient meditative practices of "circulating qi" and "standing meditation", and the slow gymnastic breathing exercise of "guiding and pulling. Traditionally, knowledge about qigong was passed from adept master to student in elite unbroken lineages, typically with secretive and esoteric traditions of training and oral transmission, and with an emphasis on meditative practice by scholars and gymnastic or dynamic practice by the working masses.

Starting in the late 1940s and the 1950s, the mainland Chinese government tried to integrate disparate qigong approaches into one coherent system, with the intention of establishing a firm scientific basis for qigong practice. In 1949, Liu Guizhen established the name "Qigong" to refer to the system of life preserving practices that he and his associates developed based on Dao yin and other philosophical traditions. This attempt is considered by some sinologists as the start of the modern or scientific interpretation of qigong. During the Great Leap Forward and the Cultural Revolution, qigong, along with other traditional Chinese medicine, was under tight control with limited access among the general public, but was encouraged in state-run rehabilitation centers and spread to universities and hospitals. After the Cultural Revolution, qigong, along with t'ai chi, was popularized as daily morning exercise practiced en masse throughout China.

Popularity of qigong grew rapidly during the Deng and Jiang eras after Mao Zedong's death in 1976 through the 1990s, with estimates of between 60 and 200 million practitioners throughout China. Along with popularity and state sanction came controversy and problems: claims of extraordinary abilities bordering on the supernatural, pseudoscience explanations to build credibility, a mental condition labeled qigong deviation, formation of cults, and exaggeration of claims by masters for personal benefit. In 1985, the state-run "National Qigong Science and Research Organization" was established to regulate the nation's qigong denominations. In 1999, in response to widespread revival of old traditions of spirituality, morality, and mysticism, and perceived challenges to State control, the Chinese government took measures to enforce control of public qigong practice, including shutting down qigong clinics and hospitals, and banning groups such as Zhong Gong and Falun Gong. Since the 1999 crackdown, qigong research and practice have only been officially supported in the context of health and traditional Chinese medicine. The Chinese Health Qigong Association, established in 2000, strictly regulates public qigong practice, with limitation of public gatherings, requirement of state approved training and certification of instructors, and restriction of practice to state-approved forms.

Through the forces of migration of the Chinese diaspora, tourism in China, and globalization, the practice of qigong spread from the Chinese community to the world. Today, millions of people around the world practice qigong and believe in the benefits of qigong to varying degrees. Similar to its historical origin, those interested in qigong come from diverse backgrounds and practice it for different reasons, including for recreation, exercise, relaxation, preventive medicine, self-healing, alternative medicine, self-cultivation, meditation, spirituality, and martial arts training.

Practices

Qigong comprises a diverse set of practices that coordinate body, breath, and mind based on Chinese philosophy. Practices include moving and still meditation, massage, chanting, sound meditation, and non-contact treatments, performed in a broad array of body postures. Qigong is commonly classified into two foundational categories: 1) dynamic or active qigong (dong gong), with slow flowing movement; and 2) meditative or passive qigong (jing gong), with still positions and inner movement of the breath. From a therapeutic perspective, qigong can be classified into two systems: 1) internal qigong, which focuses on self-care and self-cultivation, and; 2) external qigong, which involves treatment by a therapist who directs or transmits qi.

As moving meditation, qigong practice typically coordinates slow stylized movement, deep diaphragmatic breathing, and calm mental focus, with visualization of guiding qi through the body. While implementation details vary, generally qigong forms can be characterized as a mix of four types of practice: dynamic, static, meditative, and activities requiring external aids.

- Dynamic practice: Involves fluid movement, usually carefully choreographed, coordinated with breath and awareness. Examples include the slow stylized movements of T'ai chi ch'uan, Baguazhang, and Xing Yi Quan. Other examples include graceful movement that mimics the motion of animals in Five Animals (Wu Qin Xi qigong), White Crane, and Wild Goose (Dayan) Qigong. As a form of gentle exercise, qigong is composed of movements that are typically repeated, strengthening and stretching the body, increasing fluid movement (blood, synovial, and lymph), enhancing balance and proprioception, and improving the awareness of how the body moves through space.
- Static practice: Involves holding postures for sustained periods of time. In some cases this bears resemblance to the practice of Yoga and its continuation in the Buddhist tradition. For example Yiquan, a Chinese martial art derived from xingyiquan, emphasizes static stance training. In another example, the healing form Eight Pieces of Brocade (Baduanjin qigong) is based on a series of static postures.
- Meditative practice: Utilizes breath awareness, visualization, mantra, chanting, sound, and focus on philosophical concepts such as qi circulation, aesthetics, or moral values. In traditional Chinese medicine and Daoist practice, the meditative focus is commonly on cultivating qi in dantian energy centers and balancing qi flow in meridian and other pathways. In various Buddhist traditions, the aim is to still the mind, either through outward focus, for example on a place, or through inward focus on the breath, a mantra, a koan, emptiness, or the idea of the eternal. In the Confucius scholar tradition, meditation is focused on humanity and virtue, with the aim of self-enlightenment.

- Use of external agents: Many systems of qigong practice include the use of external agents such as ingestion of herbs, massage, physical manipulation, or interaction with other living organisms. For example, specialized food and drinks are used in some medical and Daoist forms, whereas massage and body manipulation are sometimes used in martial arts forms. In some medical systems a qigong master uses non-contact treatment, purportedly guiding qi through his or her own body into the body of another person.

Forms

There are numerous qigong forms. 75 ancient forms that can be found in ancient literature and also 56 common or contemporary forms have been described in a qigong compendium. The list is by no means exhaustive. Many contemporary forms were developed by people who had recovered from their illness after qigong practice.

In 2003, the Chinese Health Qigong Association officially recognized four health qigong forms:

- Muscle-Tendon Change Classic.
- Five Animals.
- Six Healing Sounds.
- Eight Pieces of Brocade.

In 2010, the Chinese Health Qigong Association officially recognized five additional health qigong forms:

- Tai Chi Yang Sheng Zhang: A tai chi form from the stick tradition.
- Shi Er Duan Jin: Seated exercises to strengthen the neck, shoulders, waist, and legs.
- Daoyin Yang Sheng Gong Shi Er Fa: 12 routines from Daoyin tradition of guiding and pulling qi.
- Mawangdui Daoyin: Guiding qi along the meridians with synchronous movement and awareness.
- Da Wu: Choreographed exercises to lubricate joints and guide qi.

Other commonly practised qigong styles and forms include:

- Soaring Crane Qigong.
- Wisdom Healing Qigong.
- Pan Gu Mystical Qigong.

- Wild Goose (Dayan) Qigong.
- Dragon and Tiger Qigong.
- Primordial Qigong (Wujigong).
- Chilel Qigong.
- Phoenix Qigong.
- Yuan Qigong.
- Zhong Yuan Qigong.

Techniques

Whether viewed from the perspective of exercise, health, philosophy, or martial arts training, several main principles emerge concerning the practice of qigong:

- Intentional movement: Careful, flowing balanced style.
- Rhythmic breathing: Slow, deep, coordinated with fluid movement.
- Awareness: Calm, focused meditative state.
- Visualization: Of qi flow, philosophical tenets, aesthetics.
- Chanting/Sound: Use of sound as a focal point.

Additional principles:

- Softness: Soft gaze, expressionless face.
- Solid Stance: Firm footing, erect spine.
- Relaxation: Relaxed muscles, slightly bent joints.
- Balance and Counterbalance: Motion over the center of gravity.

Advanced goals:

- Equanimity: More fluid, more relaxed
- Tranquility: Empty mind, high awareness
- Stillness: Smaller and smaller movements, eventually to complete stillness

The most advanced practice is generally considered to be with little or no motion.

Traditional and Classical Theory

Over time, five distinct traditions or schools of qigong developed in China, each with its own theories and characteristics: Chinese Medical Qigong, Daoist Qigong, Buddhist

Qigong, Confucian Qigong, and martial arts qigong. All of these qigong traditions include practices intended to cultivate and balance qi.

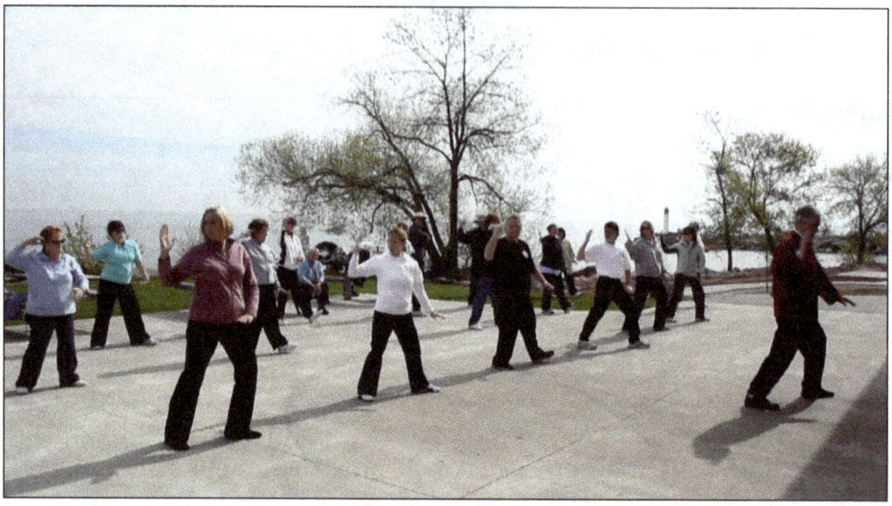

Qigong practitioners in Brazil.

Traditional Chinese Medicine

The theories of ancient Chinese qigong include the Yin-Yang and Five Phases Theory, Essence-Qi-Spirit Theory, Zang-Xiang Theory, and Meridians and Qi-Blood Theory, which have been synthesized as part of Traditional Chinese Medicine (TCM). TCM focuses on tracing and correcting underlying disharmony, in terms of deficiency and excess, using the complementary and opposing forces of yin and yang, to create a balanced flow of qi. Qi is believed to be cultivated and stored in three main dantian energy centers and to travel through the body along twelve main meridians, with numerous smaller branches and tributaries. The main meridians correspond to twelve main organs. Qi is balanced in terms of yin and yang in the context of the traditional system of Five Phases. A person is believed to become ill or die when qi becomes diminished or unbalanced. Health is believed to be returned by rebuilding qi, eliminating qi blockages, and correcting qi imbalances. These TCM concepts do not translate readily to modern science and medicine.

Daoism

In Daoism various practices now known as Daoist Qigong are claimed to provide a way to achieve longevity and spiritual enlightenment, as well as a closer connection with the natural world.

Buddhism

In Buddhism meditative practices now known as Buddhist Qigong are part of a spiritual path that leads to spiritual enlightenment or Buddhahood.

Confucianism

In Confucianism practices now known as Confucian Qigong provide a means to become a Junzi through awareness of morality.

Contemporary Qigong

In contemporary China, the emphasis of qigong practice has shifted away from traditional philosophy, spiritual attainment, and folklore, and increasingly to health benefits, traditional medicine and martial arts applications, and a scientific perspective. Qigong is now practiced by millions worldwide, primarily for its health benefits, though many practitioners have also adopted traditional philosophical, medical, or martial arts perspectives, and even use the long history of qigong as evidence of its effectiveness.

Contemporary Chinese Medical Qigong

Qigong has been recognized as a "standard medical technique" in China since 1989, and is sometimes included in the medical curriculum of major universities in China. The 2013 English translation of the official Chinese Medical Qigong textbook used in China defines CMQ as "the skill of body-mind exercise that integrates body, breath, and mind adjustments into one" and emphasizes that qigong is based on "adjustment" (tiao also translated as "regulation", "tuning", or "alignment.") of body, breath, and mind. As such, qigong is viewed by practitioners as being more than common physical exercise, because qigong combines postural, breathing, and mental training in one to produce a particular psychophysiological state of being. While CMQ is still based on traditional and classical theory, modern practitioners also emphasize the importance of a strong scientific basis. According to the 2013 CMQ textbook, physiological effects of qigong are numerous, and include improvement of respiratory and cardiovascular function, and possibly neurophysiological function.

Conventional Medicine

Conventional or mainstream medicine includes specific practices and techniques based on the best available evidence demonstrating effectiveness and safety. Qigong is not generally considered to be part of mainstream medicine, because there is no peer-reviewed scientific evidence to support the effectiveness of qigong for specific medical conditions. Similarly, there is no scientific evidence that qi (other than in its literal sense of breath) exists. Qigong is therefore not supported by modern medicine, and so, at present, there is no medical interest in Qigong.

Integrative, Complementary and Alternative Medicine

Integrative medicine (IM) refers to "the blending of conventional and complementary medicines and therapies with the aim of using the most appropriate of either or both modalities to care for the patient as a whole", whereas complementary is using a non-mainstream approach together with conventional medicine, while alternative is using a non-mainstream approach in place of conventional medicine. Qigong is used by integrative medicine practitioners to complement conventional medical treatment, based on complementary and alternative medicine interpretations of the effectiveness and safety of qigong.

Scientific Basis

Scientists interested in qigong have sought to describe or verify the effects of qigong, to explore mechanisms of effects, to form scientific theory with respect to Qigong, and to identify appropriate research methodology for further study. In terms of traditional theory, the existence of qi has not been independently verified in an experimental setting.

Health Applications

Recreation and Popular Use

People practice qigong for many different reasons, including for recreation, exercise and relaxation, preventive medicine and self-healing, meditation and self-cultivation, and training for martial arts. Practitioners range from athletes to the physically challenged. Because it is low impact and can be done lying, sitting, or standing, qigong is accessible for disabled persons, seniors, and people recovering from injuries.

Therapeutic Use

Therapeutic use of qigong is directed by TCM, CAM, integrative medicine, and other health practitioners. In China, where it is considered a "standard medical technique", qigong is commonly prescribed to treat a wide variety of conditions, and clinical applications include hypertension, coronary artery disease, peptic ulcers, chronic liver diseases, diabetes mellitus, obesity, menopause syndrome, chronic fatigue syndrome, insomnia, tumors and cancer, lower back and leg pain, cervical spondylosis, and myopia. Outside China qigong is used in integrative medicine to complement or supplement accepted medical treatments, including for relaxation, fitness, rehabilitation, and treatment of specific conditions. However, there is no high-quality evidence that qigong is actually effective for these conditions. Based on systematic reviews of clinical research, it is not possible within current level of available evidence to draw conclusions concerning effectiveness of qigong for specific medical conditions at this stage.

Safety and Cost

Qigong is generally viewed as safe. No adverse effects have been observed in clinical trials, such that qigong is considered safe for use across diverse populations. Cost for self-care is minimal, and cost efficiencies are high for group delivered care. Typically the cautions associated with qigong are the same as those associated with any physical activity, including risk of muscle strains or sprains, advisability of stretching to prevent injury, general safety for use alongside conventional medical treatments, and consulting with a physician when combining with conventional treatment.

Clinical Research

Although there is ongoing clinical research examining the potential health effects of qigong, there is little financial or medical incentive to support high-quality research, and still only a limited number of studies meet accepted medical and scientific standards of randomized controlled trials (RCTs). Clinical research concerning qigong has been conducted for a wide range of medical conditions, including bone density, cardiopulmonary effects, physical function, falls and related risk factors, quality of life, immune function, inflammation, hypertension, pain, Parkinson's disease, and cancer treatment.

A 2017 systematic review concluded that Baduanjin qigong is beneficial for quality of life, sleep quality, balance, handgrip strength, trunk flexibility, systolic and diastolic blood pressure, and resting heart rate; and that reviewed studies are insufficient to confirm benefits for leg power, cardiopulmonary endurance, and pulmonary function.

A 2015 systematic review of the effect of qigong exercises on cardiovascular diseases and hypertension found no conclusive evidence for effect, and generally poor quality of research on the potential effects of affecting blood pressure. Another systematic review found that qigong exercises improved blood pressure compared to doing nothing, but was not superior to standard treatment such as medications or conventional exercise. Another 2015 systematic review of the effect of qigong exercises on biomarkers of diabetes mellitus concluded that there was insufficient evidence for effect due to methodological problems with the underlying clinical trials.

A 2011 overview of systematic reviews of clinical trials concluded that "the effectiveness of qigong is based mostly on poor quality research" and "therefore, it would be unwise to draw firm conclusions at this stage". Although a 2010 comprehensive literature review found 77 peer-reviewed RCTs; systematic reviews for particular health conditions show that most clinical research is of poor quality, typically because of small sample size and lack of proper control groups, with lack of blinding associated with high risk of bias.

A 2010 systematic review of the effect of qigong exercises on cancer treatment concluded "the effectiveness of qigong in cancer care is not yet supported by the evidence from rigorous clinical trials." A separate systematic review that looked at the effects of qigong exercises on various physiological or psychological outcomes found that the available studies were poorly designed, with a high of bias in the results. Therefore, the authors concluded, "Due to limited number of RCTs in the field and methodological problems and high risk of bias in the included studies, it is still too early to reach a conclusion about the efficacy and the effectiveness of qigong exercise as a form of health practice adopted by the cancer patients during their curative, palliative, and rehabilitative phases of the cancer journey."

A 2009 systematic review on the effect of qigong exercises on reducing pain concluded that "the existing trial evidence is not convincing enough to suggest that internal qigong is an effective modality for pain management."

Mental Health

Many claims have been made that qigong can benefit or ameliorate mental health conditions, including improved mood, decreased stress reaction, and decreased anxiety and depression. Most medical studies have only examined psychological factors as secondary goals, although various studies have shown decreases in cortisol levels, a chemical hormone produced by the body in response to stress.

China

Basic and clinical research in China during the 1980s was mostly descriptive, and few results were reported in peer-reviewed English-language journals. Qigong became known outside China in the 1990s, and clinical randomized controlled trials investigating the effectiveness of qigong on health and mental conditions began to be published worldwide, along with systematic reviews.

Challenges

Most existing clinical trials have small sample sizes and many have inadequate controls. Of particular concern is the impracticality of double blinding using appropriate sham treatments, and the difficulty of placebo control, such that benefits often cannot be distinguished from the placebo effect. Also of concern is the choice of which qigong form to use and how to standardize the treatment or amount with respect to the skill of the practitioner leading or administering treatment, the tradition of individualization of treatments, and the treatment length, intensity, and frequency.

Meditation and Self-cultivation Applications

Qigong is practiced for meditation and self-cultivation as part of various philosophical and spiritual traditions. As meditation, qigong is a means to still the mind and enter a state of consciousness that brings serenity, clarity, and bliss. Many practitioners find qigong, with its gentle focused movement, to be more accessible than seated meditation.

Qigong for self-cultivation can be classified in terms of traditional Chinese philosophy: Daoist, Buddhist, and Confucian.

Martial Arts Applications

The practice of qigong is an important component in both internal and external style Chinese martial arts. Focus on qi is considered to be a source of power as well as the foundation of the internal style of martial arts (Neijia). T'ai Chi Ch'uan, Xing Yi Quan, and Baguazhang are representative of the types of Chinese martial arts that rely on the concept of qi as the foundation. Extraordinary feats of martial arts prowess, such as the ability to withstand heavy strikes and the ability to break hard objects are abilities attributed to qigong training.

T'ai Chi Ch'uan and Qigong

T'ai Chi Ch'uan (Taijiquan) is a widely practiced Chinese internal martial style based on the theory of taiji ("grand ultimate"), closely associated with qigong, and typically involving more complex choreographed movement coordinated with breath, done slowly for health and training, or quickly for self-defense. Many scholars consider t'ai chi ch'uan to be a type of qigong, traced back to an origin in the seventeenth century. In modern practice, qigong typically focuses more on health and meditation rather than martial applications, and plays an important role in training for t'ai chi ch'uan, in particular used to build strength, develop breath control, and increase vitality ("life energy").

References

- Ownby, david (2008). Falun gong and the future of china. Oxford: oxford university press. Isbn 978-0-19-532905-6
- Many-benefits chinese cupping-1: pacificcollege.edu, Retrieved 6 January 2020
- Crislip, mark (24 december 2014). "acupuncture odds and ends". Science-based medicine. Retrieved 8 august 2016
- Chen, b; li, my; liu, pd; guo, y; chen, zl (july 2015). "alternative medicine: an update on cupping therapy". Qjm : monthly journal of the association of physicians. 108 (7): 523–5. Doi:10.1093/qjmed/hcu227. Pmid 25399022
- singh, simon; ernst, edzard (2008). Trick or treatment. Transworld publishers. P. 368. Isbn 978-0-552-15762-9
- Gua-sha, health: healthline.com, Retrieved 13 May, 2020
- Plaugher, noel (2015). Standing qigong for health and martial arts, zhan zhuang. Ebooks corporation. Isbn 9780857012043
- Tuina takeaway, health: healthline.com, Retrieved 8 January, 2020
- Ho, peng yoke (oct 2000). Li, qi, and shu: an introduction to science and civilization in china. Dover publications. Isbn 978-0-486-41445-4

Chinese Herbal Medicine

7 CHAPTER

Chinese herbal medicine includes various remedies, herbs, therapies such as Chinese herbal therapy, Chinese patent medicine, tonifying herbs, downward draining herbs, etc. The topics elaborated in this chapter will help in gaining a better perspective of the aspects related to Chinese herbal medicine.

Chinese herbal medicine, also known as Chinese herbology is one of the primary modalities within the scope of Oriental medicine. According to the National Center for Complementary and Alternative Medicine, Oriental medicine (which includes the practice of acupuncture, Chinese herbology and Asian bodywork therapy) is a complete system of healing that dates back to 200 B.C.

Chinese herbology includes treatment with substances such as plants, roots, minerals and more. Like acupuncture, Chinese herbology has evolved as an integral part of Chinese medicine and is used to re-harmonize imbalances in the body.

Chinese formulas are comprised of herbs designed for each individual patient. This special formulation is crucial because these formulas must be delicately composed for the purpose of achieving balance in each disharmonious state of being. Even small deviations in dosage or herb composition can change the entire focus of the formula and therefore, the results.

Herbal Descriptions and Forms

The following are descriptions of herbal medicines as defined:

- Herbs are pure plant material such as leaves, flowers, fruit, seed, stems, wood, bark, roots, rhizomes or other plant parts, which may be whole, fragmented or powdered.
- Herbal Materials, like actual herbs, consist of fresh juices, gums, fixed oils, essential oils, resins and dry powders of herbs. In some countries, these materials may be processed by various local procedures such as steaming, roasting, stir-baking with honey, alcoholic beverages or other materials.
- Herbal Preparations are finished herbal products which may include pulverized or powdered herbal materials, extracts, tinctures and fatty oils of herbal materials. They also include preparations made by steeping or heating herbal materials in alcoholic beverages and/or honey, or in other materials.

- Finished Herbal Products are products made from one or more herbs. If more than one herb is used, the term herbal mixture product can also be used. Finished herbal products may contain inert substances used as a diluent or vehicle for holding the herb.
- Raw Formulas consists of carefully individually weighed unprocessed natural herbs placed together in individual bags.
- Prepared Patent Medicine is a term used for popular formulas used for generations for common illnesses. They are tiny herbal pellets which are taken two to three times daily. These are pre-formulated based on treating a specific patient problem.
- Freeze Dried Granules or Freeze Dried Pills are raw formulas cooked and freeze dried: Raw formulas are still the strongest method for taking Chinese herbs.
- Tinctures are available in prepackaged form and through special order. This method is comparable to the freeze-dried method.
- Topical Liquids and Creams are numerous and available to treat many different medical conditions such as athlete's foot, burns, hemorrhoids, bleeding, and bone problems, to name a few.

Preparation

Decoction

Typically, one batch of medicinals is prepared as a decoction of about 9 to 18 substances. Some of these are considered as main herbs, some as ancillary herbs; within the ancillary herbs, up to three categories can be distinguished. Some ingredients are added in order to cancel out toxicity or side-effects of the main ingredients; on top of that, some medicinals require the use of other substances as catalysts.

Chinese Herbal Extracts

Chinese herbal extracts are herbal decoctions that have been condensed into a granular or powdered form. Herbal extracts, similar to patent medicines, are easier and more convenient for patients to take. The industry extraction standard is 5:1, meaning for every five pounds of raw materials, one pound of herbal extract is derived.

Categorization

There are several different methods to classify traditional Chinese medicinals:

- The four natures.
- The five flavors.

- The meridians.
- The specific function.

Four Natures

The Four Natures are: hot, warm, cool cold or neutral in terms of temperature. Hot and warm herbs are used to treat cold diseases, while cool and cold herbs are used to treat heat diseases.

Five Flavors

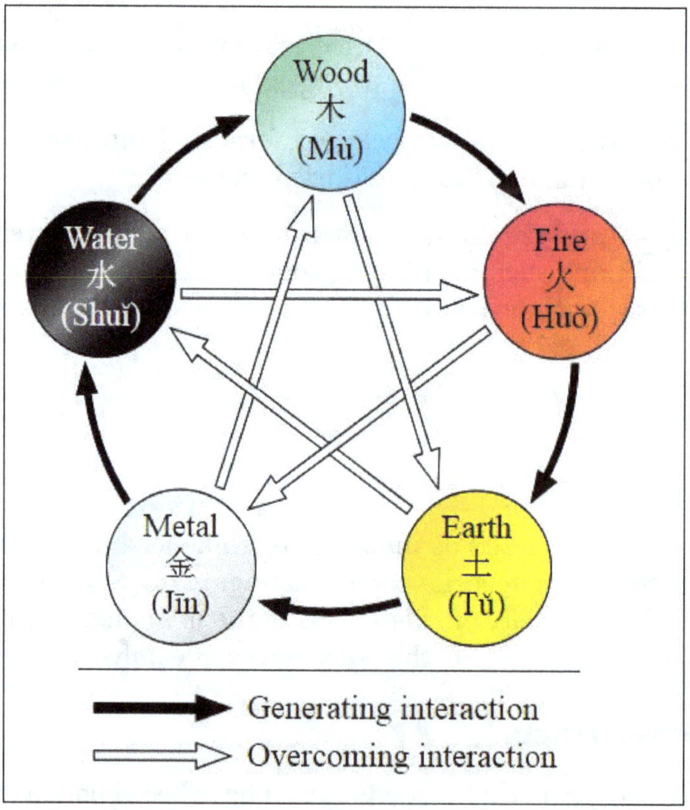

The Five Phases, which correspond to the Five Flavors.

The Five Flavors, sometimes also translated as Five Tastes, are: acrid/pungent, sweet bitter sour and salty. Substances may also have more than one flavor, or none (i.e., a bland flavor). Each of the Five Flavors corresponds to one of the zàng organs, which in turn corresponds to one of the Five Phases: A flavor implies certain properties and presumed therapeutic "actions" of a substance: saltiness "drains downward and softens hard masses"; sweetness is "supplementing, harmonizing, and moistening"; pungent substances are thought to induce sweat and act on qi and blood; sourness tends to be astringent in nature; bitterness "drains heat, purges the bowels, and eliminates dampness".

Specific Function

These categories mainly include:

- Exterior-releasing or exterior-resolving.
- Heat-clearing.
- Downward-draining or precipitating.
- Wind-damp-dispelling.
- Dampness-transforming.
- Promoting the movement of water and percolating dampness or dampness-percolating.
- Interior-warming.
- Qi-regulating or qi-rectifying.
- Dispersing food accumulation or food-dispersing.
- Worm-expelling.
- Stopping bleeding or blood-stanching.
- Quickening the Blood and dispelling stasis or blood-quickening or Blood-moving.
- Transforming phlegm, stopping coughing and calming wheezing or phlegm-transforming and cough- and panting-suppressing.
- Spirit-quieting or Shen-calming.
- Calming the Liver and expelling wind or Liver-calming and wind-extinguishing.
- Orifice-opening.
- Supplementing or tonifying: this includes qi-supplementing, blood-nourishing, yin-enriching, and yang-fortifying.
- Astriction-promoting or securing and astringing.
- Vomiting-inducing.
- Substances for external application.

Nomenclature

Many herbs earn their names from their unique physical appearance. Examples of such names include Niu Xi (Radix cyathulae seu achyranthis), "cow's knees," which has big joints that might look like cow knees; Bai Mu Er (Fructificatio tremellae fuciformis), white wood ear,' which is white and resembles an ear; Gou Ji (Rhizoma cibotii), 'dog spine,' which resembles the spine of a dog.

Color

Color is not only a valuable means of identifying herbs, but in many cases also provides information about the therapeutic attributes of the herb. For example, yellow herbs are referred to as huang (yellow) or jin (gold). Huang Bai (Cortex Phellodendri) means 'yellow fir," and Jin Yin Hua (Flos Lonicerae) has the label 'golden silver flower."

Smell and Taste

Unique flavors define specific names for some substances. Gan means 'sweet,' so Gan Cao (Radix glycyrrhizae) is 'sweet herb," an adequate description for the licorice root. "Ku" means bitter, thus Ku Shen (Sophorae flavescentis) translates as 'bitter herb.'

Geographic Location

The locations or provinces in which herbs are grown often figure into herb names. For example, Bei Sha Shen (Radix glehniae) is grown and harvested in northern China, whereas Nan Sha Shen (Radix adenophorae) originated in southern China. And the Chinese words for north and south are respectively bei and nan.

Chuan Bei Mu (Bulbus fritillariae cirrhosae) and Chuan Niu Xi (Radix cyathulae) are both found in Sichuan province, as the character "chuan" indicates in their names.

Function

Some herbs, like Fang Feng (Radix Saposhnikoviae), literally 'prevent wind," prevents or treats wind-related illnesses. Xu Duan (Radix Dipsaci), literally 'restore the broken,' effectively treats torn soft tissues and broken bones.

Country of Origin

Many herbs indigenous to other countries have been incorporated into the Chinese materia medica. Xi Yang Shen (Radix panacis quinquefolii), imported from North American crops, translates as 'western ginseng," while Dong Yang Shen (Radix ginseng Japonica), grown in and imported from North Asian countries, is 'eastern ginseng.'

Toxicity

From the earliest records regarding the use of medicinals to today, the toxicity of certain substances has been described in all Chinese materia medica. Since TCM has become more popular in the Western world, there are increasing concerns about the potential toxicity of many traditional Chinese medicinals including plants, animal parts and minerals. For most medicinals, efficacy and toxicity testing are based on traditional knowledge rather than laboratory analysis. The toxicity in some cases could be confirmed by modern research (i.e., in scorpion); in some cases it could not (i.e., in Curculigo). Further, ingredients may have different names in different locales or in historical texts, and different preparations may have similar names for the same reason, which can create inconsistencies and confusion in the creation of medicinals, with the possible danger of poisoning. Edzard Ernst "concluded that adverse effects of herbal medicines are an important albeit neglected subject in dermatology, which deserves further systematic investigation." Research suggests that the toxic heavy metals and undeclared drugs found in Chinese herbal medicines might be a serious health issue.

Substances known to be potentially dangerous include aconite, secretions from the Asiatic toad, powdered centipede, the Chinese beetle (Mylabris phalerata, Ban mao), and certain fungi. There are health problems associated with Aristolochia. Toxic effects are also frequent with Aconitum. To avoid its toxic adverse effects Xanthium sibiricum must be processed. Hepatotoxicity has been reported with products containing Reynoutria multiflora (synonym Polygonum multiflorum), glycyrrhizin, Senecio and Symphytum. The evidence suggests that hepatotoxic herbs also include Dictamnus dasycarpus, Astragalus membranaceous, and Paeonia lactiflora; although there is no evidence that they cause liver damage. Contrary to popular belief, Ganoderma lucidum mushroom extract, as an adjuvant for cancer immunotherapy, appears to have the potential for toxicity.

Also, adulteration of some herbal medicine preparations with conventional drugs which may cause serious adverse effects, such as corticosteroids, phenylbutazone, phenytoin, and glibenclamide, has been reported.

However, many adverse reactions are due to misuse or abuse of Chinese medicine. For example, the misuse of the dietary supplement Ephedra (containing ephedrine) can lead to adverse events including gastrointestinal problems as well as sudden death from cardiomyopathy. Products adulterated with pharmaceuticals for weight loss or erectile dysfunction are one of the main concerns. Chinese herbal medicine has been a major cause of acute liver failure in China.

Most Chinese herbs are safe but some have shown not to be. Reports have shown products being contaminated with drugs, toxins, or false reporting of ingredients. Some herbs used in TCM may also react with drugs, have side effects, or be dangerous to people with certain medical conditions.

Efficacy

Only a few trials exist that are considered to have adequate methodology by scientific standards. Proof of effectiveness is poorly documented or absent. A 2016 Cochrane review found "insufficient evidence that Chinese Herbal Medicines were any more or less effective than placebo or Hormonal Therapy" for the relief of menopause related symptoms. A 2012 Cochrane review found no difference in decreased mortality when Chinese herbs were used alongside Western medicine versus Western medicine exclusively. A 2010 Cochrane review found there is not enough robust evidence to support the effectiveness of traditional Chinese medicine herbs to stop the bleeding from haemorrhoids. A 2008 Cochrane review found promising evidence for the use of Chinese herbal medicine in relieving painful menstruation, compared to conventional medicine such as NSAIDs and the oral contraceptive pill, but the findings are of low methodological quality. A 2012 Cochrane review found weak evidence suggesting that some Chinese medicinal herbs have a similar effect at preventing and treating influenza as antiviral medication. Due to the poor quality of these medical studies, there is insufficient evidence to support or dismiss the use of Chinese medicinal herbs for the treatment of influenza. There is a need for larger and higher quality randomized clinical trials to determine how effective Chinese herbal medicine is for treating people with influenza. A 2005 Cochrane review found that although the evidence was weak for the use of any single herb, there was low quality evidence that some Chinese medicinal herbs may be effective for the treatment of acute pancreatitis.

Successful results have been scarce: artemisinin is one of few examples. An effective treatment for malaria, it was derived from Artemisia annua which is traditionally used to treat fever. Chinese herbology is largely pseudoscience, with no valid mechanism of action for the majority of its treatments.

Ecological Impacts

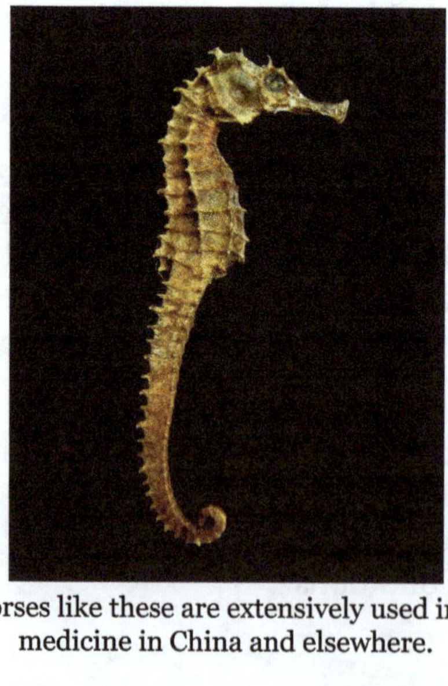

Dried seahorses like these are extensively used in traditional medicine in China and elsewhere.

The traditional practice of using (by now) endangered species is controversial within TCM. Modern Materia Medicas such as Bensky, Clavey and Stoger's comprehensive

Chinese herbal text discuss substances derived from endangered species in an appendix, emphasizing alternatives.

Parts of endangered species used as TCM drugs include tiger bones and rhinoceros horn. Poachers supply the black market with such substances, and the black market in rhinoceros horn, for example, has reduced the world's rhino population by more than 90 percent over the past 40 years. Concerns have also arisen over the use of turtle plastron and seahorses.

TCM recognizes bear bile as a medicinal. In 1988, the Chinese Ministry of Health started controlling bile production, which previously used bears killed before winter. Now bears are fitted with a sort of permanent catheter, which is more profitable than killing the bears. More than 12,000 asiatic black bears are held in "bear farms", where they suffer cruel conditions while being held in tiny cages. The catheter leads through a permanent hole in the abdomen directly to the gall bladder, which can cause severe pain. Increased international attention has mostly stopped the use of bile outside of China; gallbladders from butchered cattle (niú dǎn) are recommended as a substitute for this ingredient.

Collecting American ginseng to assist the Asian traditional medicine trade has made ginseng the most harvested wild plant in North America for the last two centuries, which eventually led to a listing on CITES Appendix II.

Herbs in Use

Chinese herbology is a pseudoscientific practice with potentially unreliable product quality, safety hazards or misleading health advice. There are regulatory bodies, such as China GMP (Good Manufacturing Process) of herbal products. However, there have been notable cases of an absence of quality control during herbal product preparation. There is a lack of high-quality scientific research on herbology practices and product effectiveness for anti-disease activity. In the herbal sources listed below, there is little or no evidence for efficacy or proof of safety across consumer age groups and disease conditions for which they are intended.

There are over 300 herbs in common use. Some of the most commonly used herbs are Ginseng rénshēn), wolfberry dong quai (Angelica sinensis, dāngguī), astragalus huángqí), atractylodes báizhú), bupleurum cháihú), cinnamon (cinnamon twigs (guìzhī) and cinnamon bark (ròuguì)), coptis (huánglián), ginger (jiāng), hoelen (fúlíng), licorice (gāncǎo), ephedra sinica (máhuáng), peony (white: báisháo and reddish: chìsháo), rehmannia (dìhuáng), rhubarb (dàhuáng), and salvia (dānshēn).

Chinese Ginseng

The use of Chinese ginseng is well over 2,000 years old in Chinese medicine. The constituents include steroid saponins known as ginsenosides, The amount of ginsenosides in Chinese ginseng depends on how the plant was cultivated and the age of the root. Wild Chinese ginseng, believed to be of highest TCM quality, has become rare in its natural habitat, so natural fostering efforts are utilized to emulate the wild variety. Chinese ginseng can be white or red, depending on how it is processed. White Chinese ginseng is unprocessed and dried naturally. Red Chinese ginseng is processed with steam and, in TCM, is believed to be more potent.

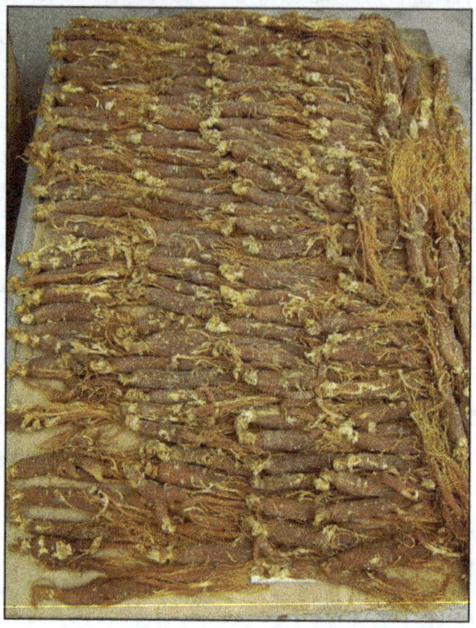

Chinese red ginseng roots.

- TCM Lore.
- Properties: Sweet, Bitter, Warm.
- Channels: Lung, Spleen, Heart.

American Ginseng

Wild American ginseng populations are thought to be less abundant than they were in the 18th and early 19th centuries, due to habitat loss, harvest pressures and excessive deer browse. Current American ginseng products are commonly sourced from naturally fostered varieties, to emulate the wild variety.

- TCM Lore.
- Properties: Sweet, Slightly Bitter, Cold.
- Channels: Heart, Kidney, Lung.

Siberian Ginseng

- TCM Lore.
- Properties: Pungent, Acrid, Slightly Bitter, Warm.
- Channels: Spleen, Heart, Kidney.

Ginkgo

Mushrooms

Mushrooms have long been used as a medicinal food and as a tea in Chinese herbology.

Wolfberry

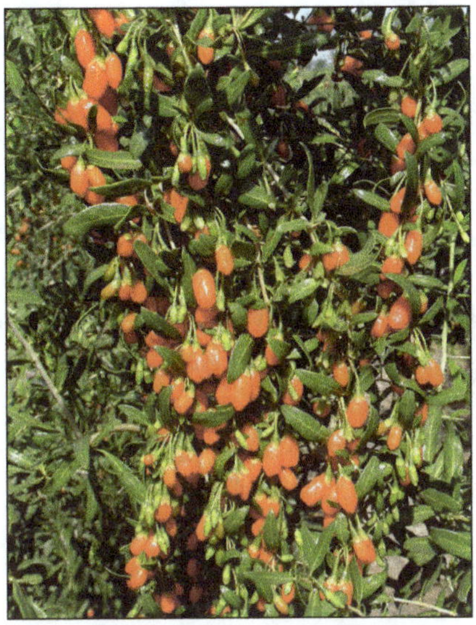

Lycium barbarum, Wolfberry.

Wolfberry is grown in Ningxia from shrubs with long vines. The shrubs are covered with small trumpet-shaped flowers, which turn into small, bright red berries. The berries are usually consumed fresh and sometimes when dried.

Dang Gui

Dang Gui (Angelica sinensis or "female ginseng") is an aromatic herb that grows in China, Korea, and Japan.

- Species: Angelica sinensis.
- Pinyin: Dang Gui.
- Common Name: Chinese Angelica Root.
- Quality: Sweet, Pungent (Acrid), Warm.
- Meridians: Liver, Heart, Spleen.

Astragalus

Astragalus is a root.

- Species: Astragalus membranaceus.

- Pinyin: Huang Qi.
- Common Name: Astragalus Root, Milkvetch Root.
- Quality: Sweet, Slightly warm.
- Meridians: Lung, Spleen.

Atractylodes

- Species: Atractylodes lancea.
- Pinyin: Cang Zhu.
- Common Name: Atractylodes Rhizome.
- Quality: Pungent (Acrid), Bitter, Warm.
- Meridians: Spleen, Stomach.

Bupleurum

- Species: Bupleurum chinense.
- Pinyin: Chai Hu.
- Common Name: Hare's Ear Root.
- Quality: Bitter, Pungent (Acrid), Cool.
- Meridians: Gallbladder, Liver, Pericardium, San Jiao.

Cinnamon

Cinnamon, mostly gui zhi and rou gui, is the twigs and bark from a species of large tropical tree.

- Species: Cinnamomum cassia.
- Pinyin: Gui Zhi.
- Common Name: Cinnamon Twig.
- Quality: Pungent (Acrid), Sweet, Warm.
- Meridians: Heart, Lung, Bladder.
- Species: Cinnamomum cassia.
- Pinyin: Rou Gui.

- Common Name: Cinnamon Bark.
- Quality: Pungent (Acrid), Sweet, Hot.
- Meridians: Heart, Kidney, Liver, Spleen.

Coptis Chinensis

The rhizome of Coptis chinensis is one of the bitterest herbs used in Chinese medicine.

- Species: Coptis chinensis.
- Pinyin: Huang Lian.
- Common Name: Coptis Rhizome.
- Qualities: Bitter, Cold.
- Meridians: Heart, Large Intestine, Liver, Stomach.

Ginger

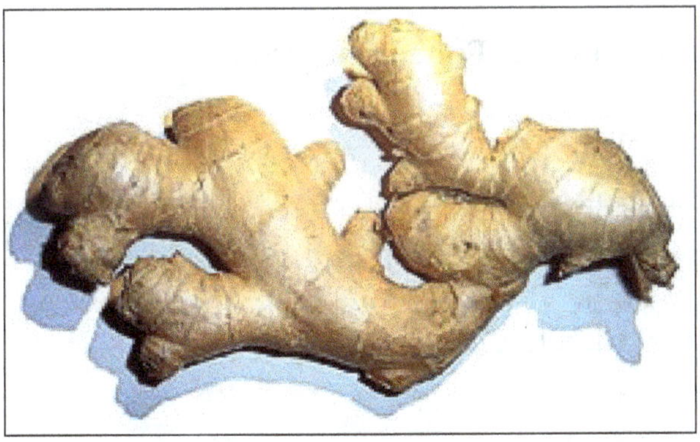

Ginger is consumed in China as food and as medicine.

Ginger is a herb and a spice that is used in Chinese cuisine. There are four main kinds of preparations in Chinese herbology: fresh ginger, dried ginger, roasted ginger, and ginger charcoal, all made of the rhizomes.

- Species: Zingiber officinalis.
- Pinyin: Sheng Jiang.
- Common Name: Fresh Ginger Rhizome.
- Quality: Pungent (Acrid), Slightly warm.
- Meridians: Lung, Spleen, Stomach.
- Species: Zingiber officinalis.

- Pinyin: Gan Jiang.
- Common Name: Dried Ginger Rhizome.
- Quality: Pungent (Acrid), Hot.
- Meridians: Heart, Lung, Spleen, Stomach.

Licorice

- Species: Glycyrrhiza inflata or Glycyrrhiza glabra.
- Pinyin: Gan Cao.
- Common Name: Licorice Root.
- Quality: Sweet, Neutral.
- Meridians: All 12 channels, but mainly Heart, Lung, Spleen, Stomach.

Ephedra

- Species: Ephedra sinica or Ephedra intermedia.
- Pinyin: Ma Huang.
- Common Name: Ephedra Stem.
- Quality: Pungent (Acrid), Slightly Bitter, Warm.
- Meridians: Lung, Bladder.

Peony

Peony comes in two varieties: bai shao ("bai"=white) and chi shao ("chi"=red). the root of the plant is used in both varieties.

- Species: Paeonia lactiflora.
- Pinyin: Bai Shao.
- Common Name: White Peony Root.
- Quality: Bitter, Sour, Cool.
- Meridians: Liver, Spleen.
- Species: Paeonia lactiflora or Paeonia veitchii.
- Pinyin: Chi Shao.

- Common Name: Red Peony Root.
- Quality: Sour, Bitter, Cool.
- Meridians: Liver, Spleen.

Rehmannia

Rehmannia is a root where the dark, moist part of the herb is used.

- Species: Rehmannia glutinosa.
- Pinyin: Sheng Di Huang.
- Common Name: Raw Chinese Foxglove Root.
- Qualities: Sweet, Bitter, Cold.
- Meridians: Heart, Kidney, Liver.
- Species: Rehmannia glutinosa.
- Pinyin: Shu Di Huang.
- Common Name: Chinese Foxglove Root Prepared with Wine.
- Qualities: Sweet, Slightly warm.
- Meridians: Heart, Kidney, Liver.

Rhubarb

Rhubarb used medicinally for its root, was one of the first herbs to be exported from China.

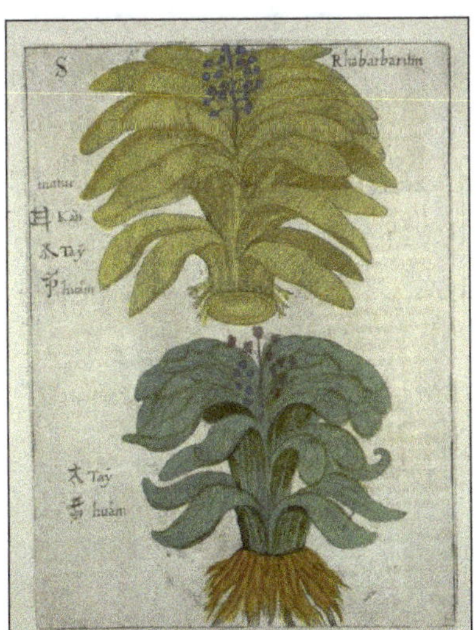

Chinese rhubarb depicted by Michał Boym.

- Species: Rheum palmatum, Rheum ranguticum, or Rheum officinale.
- Pinyin: Da Huang.
- Common Name: Rhubarb Root and Rhizome.
- Quality: Bitter, Cold.
- Meridians: Heart, Large Intestine, Liver, Stomach.

Salvia

Salvia are the deep roots of the Chinese sage plant.

- Species: Salvia miltiorrhiza.
- Pinyin: Dan Shen.
- Common Name: Salvia Root.
- Qualities: Bitter, Cool.
- Meridians: Heart, Pericardium, Liver.

CHINESE HERBAL THERAPY

Herbal therapy is important in traditional Chinese medicine. It has been used for centuries in China, where herbs are considered fundamental therapy for many acute and chronic conditions. Like acupuncture, Chinese herbs can address unhealthy body patterns that manifest in a variety of symptoms and complaints. The aims of Chinese herbal therapy are to help you regain balance in your body and to strengthen your body's resistance to disease. Chinese herbs may be used to:

- Decrease cold/flu symptoms.
- Increase your energy.
- Improve your breathing.
- Improve digestion.
- Improve your sleep.
- Decrease pain.
- Improve menopausal symptoms.
- Help regulate menstrual cycles (if infertility is an issue).

Chinese herbal therapy can also be valuable following cancer treatment to aid the body's recovery from the after-effects of chemotherapy and/or radiation. Chinese herbs are useful in the rehabilitation from many chronic diseases, as well. Chinese herbal therapy may be recommended when you have multiple symptoms or symptoms that are hard to pinpoint, or if you have exhausted traditional medical options and nothing seems to help. Chinese herbal medicine may also be useful when you need therapy to counteract side effects of prescription medications. Finally, Chinese herbal therapy is beneficial as preventive medicine.

CHINESE PATENT MEDICINE

Chinese patent medicine are herbal medicines in Traditional Chinese medicine, modernized into a ready-to-use form such as tablets, oral solutions or dry suspensions, as opposed to herbs that require cooking (hot water extraction).

Chinese patent medicines generally consist of extracted condensed pills called teapills, and are usually small, spherical, and black. They are called teapills because the herbs are cooked into an herbal tea to make the pills. Honey or water pills made from ground raw herbs are also a popular format in China, and they tend to be larger and are slightly to significantly softer than teapills.

Modern teapills are created from herbs extracted in stainless steel extractors to create either a water decoction or water-alcohol decoction, depending on the herbs used. They are extracted at a low temperature (below 100 degrees Celsius) to preserve essential ingredients. The extracted liquid is then further condensed and a small amount of raw herb powder from one of the herbal ingredients is mixed in to form an herbal dough. This dough is then cut into tiny pieces by a machine, and a small amount of excipients are added for a smoother and a more consistent exterior. The products are then made as pills.

Honey pills and water pills have been made since ancient times by combining several dried herbs and other ingredients, which are grounded into powder, mixed with a binder and traditionally formed into pills by hand. Modern honey or water pills are formed into pills by machine. The binder is traditionally honey for honey pills. For water pills the binder may simply be water, or may include another binder, such as molasses. Modern manufacturers still produce many patent formulas as honey or water pills, such as Wuji Baifeng Wan, a popular honey pill formula to "nourish qi and blood", to strengthen the body.

Patents may come in other forms such as dripping pills, liquids, syrups, powders, granules, instant teas, and capsules. Companies make Chinese patent medicines both within and outside China.

Like other patent medicines, they are not patented in the traditional sense of the word. No one has exclusive rights to the formula. Instead, "patent" refers to the standardization of the formula.

In China, all Chinese patent medicines of the same name have the same proportions of ingredients, and are manufactured in accordance with the PRC Pharmacopoeia's monograph on that particular formula, which is mandated by Chinese law. Each monograph details the exact herbal ingredients that make up the patent formula, usually accompanied by the specific tests that should be used for correct herb identification, such as thin layer chromatography (TLC) or high performance liquid chromatography (HPLC), the percentage of each ingredient, and specific cautions and contraindications. The monograph also details the manufacturing methods that must be followed, how to process and cook the herbs, often including specific requirements for finished product testing including authenticating and assessing the potency of the formula with active ingredient markers where known, as well as testing for dissolution time and content uniformity. All good manufacturing practice (GMP) certified factories must also test for heavy metal levels and microbials for all patent medicines they produce.

However, many patents do not list all ingredients, presumably to protect the secrecy of the formula. An example of this is Yunnan Baiyao, a popular formula used to stop bleeding, whose ingredients have never been revealed. This is an acceptable practice in China, where no other protection exists to protect family or "secret" Chinese herbal formulas.

In western countries, there is considerable variation of ingredients and in the proportions of ingredients in products sharing the same name. This is because the Chinese government allows foreign companies to apply for modifications of patent formulas to be sold outside of China. For example, Hebei brand Lifei pills contain Kadsura (feng sha teng) and Morus (sang ye), whereas Plum Flower brand Li Fei Pian contains Schizandra (we wei zi) and Gecko (ge jie) instead. Another example is Qing Qi Hua Tan Wan. The Lanzou brand uses Citrus (ju hong). The Lanzhou Foci Min Shan brand and the Plum Flower brand do not, but use Ginger (sheng jiang).

Herbal Formulas

Chinese classic herbal formulas form the basis of Chinese patent medicine. These are the basic herbal formulas that students of traditional Chinese medicine learn. Many of these formulas are quite old. For example, "Liu Wei Di Huang Wan" was developed by Qian Yi (c. 1032–1113 CE). It was published in the "Xiao'er Yao Zheng Zhi Jue" (also known as "Key to Therapeutics of Children's Diseases" xiǎoér yào zhèng zhí jué) in 1119 by Qian Yi's student. Although Liu Wei Di Huang Wan can be prepared as a raw herb decoction (or herbal tea), it was originally created to be made into honey pills. The last word in Liu Wei Di Huang Wan, "Wan" means "pill".

Criticisms

Heavy Metal Contamination

Some Chinese patent medicines were tested and found to contain high to dangerous levels of heavy metals. The most common heavy metals found were mercury, lead, and arsenic. These ingredients can cause serious medical problems.

Pharmaceutical Adulterants

Some Chinese patent medicines were found to contain pharmaceutical drugs such as decongestants, analgesics or antihistamines. The most common Chinese patent medicines found to carry pharmaceutical drugs were for the treatment of asthma, pain, and arthritis.

Many contaminants and drug adulterants named in the context of herbal medicine is intentionally added and declared on product labels. The mercury salt cinnabar (Chinese:pinyin: zhūshā), the arsenic salt realgar (Chinese: pinyin: xíong hung) and the strychnine containing Strychnos nux-vomica (Chinese:pinyin: Mǎqiánzǐ) are used traditionally and kept in China despite the known harm and little proven benefit.

In the case of drugs, the entry for "Vitamin C/Lonicera/Forsythia tablet" (Chinese: C pinyin: Wéi C Yínqiào Piàn) in the Chinese Pharmacopoeia (ChP) calls for 105 mg of paracetamol and 1.05 mg of chlorpheniramine maleate each pill. Such a combination is common for Chinese cold medicine. In a more hidden case, the herb Ephedra naturally contains ephedrine and pseudoephedrine, and is required by the ChP to have more than 0.8% of the two decongestants (as hydrochloride salts) in its dry weight.

Prohibited Ingredients

Some Chinese patent medicines contain ingredients which are banned in other countries. The two most common prohibited herbs are Ma Huang (má huáng) (Ephedra) and Ban Xia (bàn xià) (Pinellia). On 30 December 2003, the FDA in the US announced a ban (effective 12 April 2004), on these herbs from all dietary supplements. Traditional Chinese herbal remedies are exempt from this law.

TONIFYING HERBS

From the perspective of Traditional Chinese Medicine (TCM), an imbalance of Yin and Yang is implicated in most if not all of the diseases plaguing contemporary society. TCM practitioners attempt to correct this imbalance through tonification. Tonification is one of the eight recognized methods of herbal therapy. Specifically, it is an herbal therapeutic treatment used in those instances where there is a need to nourish and rebuild the qi (pronounced Chi) or life-energy of the body's organs and organ systems when they suffer from a deficiency or weakness or otherwise when the body's Yin and Yang are out of balance.

According to Tierra, herbs can be used as tonics to build and sustain the energy of the organ systems. Within the Eastern paradigm of medicine (e.g., Ayurveda, TCM & Tibetan medicine), herbal tonics are used to practice preventative medicine and to assist in the treatment of acute ailments and build strength when recovering from an illness, all of which is achieved by restoring and balancing energy levels or qi of the body.

Health and Wellness Monthly provides a proposed whole body tonic made-up of specific herbs designed to help bring the body's Yin and Yang back into balance and, thereby, assist in restoring and maintaining overall health after suffering from a disruption and depletion of the body's vital energy due to an illness. However, the proposed formula could be used as a preventative measure to sustain balance and vitality.

Yin and Yang Herbal Tonics

There are specific Yin and Yang herbal tonics. On the one hand, Yin-tonics feed the organs, providing them with necessary nutrients. Tierra asserts that the most valuable Yin-tonics are the "seaweeds (kelp and Irish Moss), alfalfa, comfrey and dandelion leaf". On the other hand, Yang-tonics balance and stimulate the life-energy of the organs, thereby, improving their assimilation and utilization of nutrients. According to Tierra, Chinese root tonic herbs, burdock, dandelion root, parsley, Oregon grape root and goldenseal root are considered to be among the more efficacious Yang-tonics.

Mowrey recommends the following combination of herbs to serve as a whole body tonic: Sarsaprarilla root, siberian ginseng, fo-ti, gotu kola, saw palmetto berries, licorice root, kelp, stillingia, alfalfa and cayenne.

Herbal Tonification Formula

Purpose of the Formula

Within the context of TCM and taking cues from Tierra and Mowrey, the proposed whole body tonic is intended to help provide the organs of the body with vital nutrients (Yin function support) and ensure the proper functioning of the organs (Yang function support), thereby, keeping the body's polarities of Yin and Yang in balance, while rebuilding the life-energy of the body's organs and organ systems when they suffer from deficiency or weakness or excess for that matter.

Herbs Constituting the Formula

The proposed formula would consist of kelp, alfalfa, dandelion leaf (i.e., Yin-tonic herbs), along with dandelion root, burdock, parsley, goldenseal root and siberian ginseng (i.e., Yang-tonic herbs).

Kelp (Laminaria, macrocystis, ascophyllum): This is an important herb in providing nutrients. It is recognized as general nutritive tonic. Kelp is especially rich in iodine, which assists in proper glandular function, regulation of energy and metabolism by the burning of fat. Kelp is an excellent source of vitamins A, B1, B2, C, D and E. It also contains minerals such as iron, sodium, phosphorus and calcium, magnesium and potassium. Amino acids are contained in Kelp as well.

Kelp contains properties to help improve cardiovascular function, circulation, blood pressure, nerve and gland function and thyroid function. It is also noted for helping in detoxification of the body, weight loss and fighting the inflammation associated with arthritis, among other health benefits.

Alfalfa (Medicago sativa): Alfalfa contains high amounts of vitamins A, B1 (thiamine), B6 (pyridoxine), B12 (cobalamin), C, D, E and K, along with B3 (niacin), B5 (pantothenic acid), B7 (biotin), B9 (folic acid). It also contains calcium, magnesium, chlorophyll, phosphorous, iron, potassium, zinc and copper and digestive enzymes. Alfalfa is a good source of protein. It contains saponins. Alfalfa is useful in fighting arthritis, high cholesterol and providing overall vitality and vigor. Because of its fiber content, it is effective in cellular detoxification.

Dandelion leaf (Taraxacum officinale): Dandelion leaf contains substantial levels of vitamins A, C, D, and B complex. It also contains iron, magnesium, zinc, potassium, manganese, copper, chlorine, calcium, boron, and silicon. Dandelion leaf functions as a blood purifying herb, mild laxative, diuretic to help remove toxins, digestive aid, bile production agent and liver support herb.

Dandelion root (Taraxacum officinale): Dandelion root is considered to be stronger in its metabolic action and possessing more Yang qualities than dandelion leaf. The following vitamins and minerals are contained in dandelion root: Vitamins A, C, D, riboflavin, thiamine calcium, magnesium, potassium and iron. Dandelion root is noted especially for its benefit to the liver and its elimination of toxins from the blood. It promotes the production of bile, modulates bile duct inflammation and liver congestion. Dandelion root is recognized in clearing obstructions of the spleen, pancreas, gallbladder, bladder and kidneys. Furthermore, it possesses the ability to decrease blood glucose levels, modulate the growth of harmful bacteria, provide relief from indigestion and heartburn, remove foreign particles from the gallbladder, help the gallbladder release bile for digestion and absorption of nutrients.

Burdock root (Arctium lappa): Burdock Root is a good source of vitamins A, B complex, C and E. It contains relatively high amounts of chromium, cobalt, iron, magnesium, phosphorus, potassium, silicon, and zinc. Burdock root also contains calcium, copper, manganese, selenium, and sulphur. It is a good source of the carbohydrate, inulin. Burdock root is recognized to be an effective blood purifier (i.e., alterative), diuretic and diaphoretic, all of which gives it the ability to help cleanse the body of toxins and wastes. It is associated with proven restorative effects on the liver and gallbladder. It is known as having special value in preventing and remedying disease and recuperating from sickness.

Parsley (Petroselinum sativum): Although it used frequently as garnish decorating one sort of dish or another, parsley is highly nutritive in nature and possesses various medicinal properties to help create and sustain overall health. For example, parsley is rich in vitamins and minerals, including Vitamins, A, C and K. It is a good source of the B-vitamins. In terms of minerals, parsley contains calcium, magnesium, manganese, potassium, zinc and iron. It is also contains contain up to 25% protein.

Parsley is considered to provide chemoprotective qualities, antibacterial action, anti-oxidant properties, cardiovascular protection and rheumatoid arthritis protection.

Siberian ginseng (Eleutherococcus senticosus): As a Yang tonic, siberian ginseng is recognized for its ability to enhance circulation, boost the immune system, increase energy levels, increase endurance and eliminate fatigue and low vitality by supporting the function of the adrenal glands, spleen and pancreas.

Goldenseal root (Hydrastis canadensis): Goldenseal root is recognized as a broad spectrum herb containing, Vitamins A, C, E, B-complex, calcium, iron, manganese, among other nutrients. It possesses antibiotic, anti-inflammatory and astringent properties. Goldenseal can sooth irritated mucous membranes and provide relief from excess mucous build-up in the eyes, ears, nose and throat. It has the ability to cleanse and support healthy glandular function by increasing bile and digestive enzymes.

Chinese medicine has taught for thousands of years that health is a state of balance and ill-health is an imbalance of the opposing energy forces of Yin and Yang. Readers in need of nourishing and rebuilding the qi or life-energy of his/her organs and organ systems because they suffer from deficiency or weakness or otherwise have an imbalance of Yin and Yang might want to consider using an herbal therapeutic treatment to tonify the body such as the one proposed above. The proposed formula whole body herbal tonic formula is intended to help restore and maintain overall health and balance by providing nourishment to the organs so as to improve their function.

If the reader has sufficient knowledge and training in herbology and knows how to prepare herbs to put into a formula, then he/she can prepare the formula outlined above to tonify the body. If the reader does not have such knowledge and skill, then he/she can search the internet or visit his/her local health store to purchase a formula that would contain most of the herbs in the proposed formula. It is also possible that a supplement manufacturer has put together a wholly different herbal formula to tonify the body that would help to tonify the body.

Another alternative would be to seek out the services of a professional herbalist who could put the formula together using a particular delivery system such as capsules with appropriate dosage levels of the individual herbs contained in the proposed whole body tonic. The herbalist might even recommend a different combination of herbs to tonify the body.

Whether or not readers use the exact proposed formula is not as important as it is that they acquire a whole body tonic for restoring and maintaining health and vitality if they are in need of such a tonic. Further, it is hoped that this month's newsletter serves to inform readers not familiar with the healing power of herbs and to remind those who are how herbs can be used to restore balance and vitality to the body through tonification, especially when suffering from deficiency and weakness.

HERBS TO CURE EXTERIOR SYNDROME

The term Exterior syndrome indicates, in a broad sense, that the pathogenic change is in the superficial layer of the body. The main characteristic of this change is the conflict between the six exogenous pathogenic factors and the body's resistance, which is represented mainly by the Defensive Qi in the superficial layer of the body. An Exterior syndrome also includes further pathogenic changes of the associated organs, meridians, Qi and Blood.

The Lung is an important organ in Exterior syndrome because it governs the Exterior by dispersing the Defensive Qi to the superficial layer of the body. Moreover, Wind-Heat and Dryness can directly disturb the function of the Lung because they can invade the body through the nose, and not the superficial level.

The main symptoms can be divided into two groups. On the one hand, chills, fever and aversion to cold or wind are present. These are the manifestations in the superficial layer of the body caused by the conflict between pathogenic factors and the Defensive Qi. On the other hand, headache, general pain, thirst, blocked nose, cough and sore throat may be present; these are manifestations caused by disharmony of the circulation of the Qi and Blood in the Bladder meridian and dysfunction of the Lung-Qi.

The purpose of treatment is to expel the exogenous pathogenic factors, and to restore the normal functioning and harmony of all the organs, meridians, Qi and Blood. Methods that can stimulate or strengthen the function of the Defensive Qi or disperse the Lung-Qi and therefore eliminate the pathogenic factors are often used. Other methods, such as promoting Qi and Blood circulation, or regulating the Large Intestine in order to regulate the Lung-Qi, can also be used as assistant procedures in the whole treatment strategy.

Herbs that release the Exterior have the functions of expelling Wind-Cold or Wind-Heat. They are used in conditions where the pathogenic Wind-Cold or Wind-Heat invades the superficial layer of the body. They have the following properties.

Pungent or Pungent and Warm

Most of the herbs in this category possess a pungent property. As pungency has a dispersing capacity, the pungent herbs are able to activate Qi movement, open the pores and subcutaneous layer, connect the Exterior with the Interior, disperse the Lung-Qi, harmonize the Nutritive and Defensive systems and therefore expel Wind. Moreover, many of the herbs are pungent and warm in nature. Their functions of activating the Yang and Qi and opening the pores are represented by their induction of sweating in different degrees. Through sweating, Wind and other exogenous pathogenic factors can be eliminated from the superficial layer of the body, therefore stopping the progress of the disease in its primary stage.

Aromatic

Many of the herbs in this category are aromatic, which gives them the ability to open the orifices, penetrate turbidity, spread the pure Qi and transform Dampness. They are therefore used to treat headache, dizziness, nasal obstruction and loss of the sense of smell.

Light in Weight and Gentle in Nature

Many herbs in this category are light in weight and gentle in nature. They mainly enter the Lung and the Bladder meridians, so they are suitable for treating the external pathogenic syndromes that mainly affect those layers and meridians. As wind characteristically attacks the upper body, which includes the head, the Lung, the Upper Jiao and the superficial layer of the body, these herbs are often used to treat symptoms such as headache, dizziness, nasal obstruction, runny nose, itchy and painful eyes, cough with or without production, sore throat and general body pain. Many are also used to treat allergies such as hay fever and asthma, as well as many kinds of skin diseases.

What Precautions should be Observed in the usage of Herbs that Release the Exterior?

First of all, since herbs that release the Exterior are pungent and their tendencies of action are ascending and dispersing, especially with the herbs that can cause sweating, overdose may disperse the Qi too much, consume the Yin of the body and cause other complications. In patients who are deficient in Yin or Qi owing to their constitution, chronic disease, stress or dietary habit, these herbs should be used with caution. Furthermore, as pungency also has the property of movement, these herbs should also be used with caution in bleeding conditions or in pregnancy.

Secondly, the dosage of herbs should be adjusted to suit the condition of the individual, the syndrome and the season. For elderly people, children, people with a weak constitution and for mild syndromes, in a gentle climate and in the summer, the dosage should be reduced. For adults with a strong constitution and for severe syndromes, in a cold winter or a cold place, the dosage should be increased. If sweating must be induced, the dosage is adjusted according to the syndrome. A mild sweat over the whole body is required. Heavy sweating must be avoided because it can only weaken the Qi and Yin.

In the third place, as eliminating Wind-Cold or Wind-Heat is not generally difficult, these herbs should not be used for a long period of time. A dosage of 3 days is recommended to treat Exterior syndrome. If the exogenous pathogenic factors have not been removed completely, then another 3-day dosage can be prescribed. With regard to herbs that may cause heavy sweating, the dosage and treatment course should be adjusted according to the reaction of the patient after each use.

Ma Huang and Gui Zhi

Ma Huang is also called Sheng Ma Huang. 'S heng' means 'raw'. Sheng Ma Huang is very pungent and warm. It is a very strong herb used to expel Wind and Cold to release Exterior Wind-Cold syndrome. As Sheng Ma Huang is pungent and hot, the dosage should be controlled and it should not be used over a long period of time. Overdose may cause heavy sweating, which injures the Yin, Body Fluids and Qi. It should be used with caution, especially in patients with a weak constitution and Deficiency syndrome. As its actions have an upward and outward tendency, Ma Huang should not be used or used with caution in cases of hypertension and heart disease.

Zhi Ma Huang is gentler in action compared with Sheng Ma Huang, because roasting with honey moderates the pungent taste. Zhi Ma Huang acquires the nature of honey, which is sweet and moistening, so its dispersing action is not as strong and quick as that of Sheng Ma Huang. It is often used to disperse the Lung-Qi and cause it to descend, to moisten the Lung and stop wheezing. In clinical practice, it is often used for treating asthma, bronchitis, pneumonia and acute nephritis.

Ma Huang Gen has completely different characteristics from both Sheng Ma Huang and Zhi Ma Huang. It is neutral, sweet and astringent, and enters the Lung meridian. It is excellent for stopping sweating. It can be used for treating spontaneous sweating and night sweating. It treats only the symptoms however, so it is often combined with other herbs that treat the cause of sweating. In addition, it should not be used in the syndrome of Phlegm accumulation or Exterior syndrome because it has an astringent property, which can retain Phlegm, close the pores and retain the pathogenic factors within the body.

Characteristic Functions of Gui Zhi (Cinnamomi Cassiae Ramulus)

'Twig of plants enters the limbs of human body': such similes and allegories were often used in ancient times in Chinese medicine to explain the complicated links between the human and the natural environment. Gui Zhi is an example of this. This herb is the twig of the plant and has a warm, pungent and sweet nature. Besides expelling Wind and Cold to treat Exterior syndrome, Gui Zhi is often used to treat Bi syndrome. In this case, it can relieve pain and cold sensations in the affected limbs or joints. The therapeutic effects are achieved by warming and strengthening the Heart-Yang, promoting the Blood circulation, spreading the Yang-Qi and unblocking the meridians, especially in the limbs. This is why it is often used in Bi syndrome caused by blockage of the circulation of Qi and Blood by Wind, Dampness or Cold; examples are rheumatic fever, rheumatoid arthritis, rheumatic heart disease, Raynaud's disease and the early and mid phases of vasculitis.

In chronic diseases, when internal Cold blocks the meridians, a small amount (about 10 m) of Gui Zhi alcohol drink is also a preferred formulation for daily use in the diet. Soaking 15 grams of Gui Zhi in a liter of alcohol (about 40% alcohol) made from cereals for 6 weeks yields Gui Zhi alcohol drink. Alcohol is pungent and warm, so is considered to have the functions of invigorating the Blood and unblocking the meridians. The functions of Gui Zhi and alcohol therefore enhance each other. It is commonly used for chronic Bi syndrome.

As Gui Zhi is pungent and warm, it should be used with caution if there is any deficiency of Yin with Empty-Fire or Liver-Yang rising in the syndrome or in the treatment of Heat-type Bi syndrome.

Jing Jie and Fang Feng

Jing Jie and Fang Feng are both pungent and warm. However, they are far gentler than Ma Huang and Gui Zhi. They can expel Wind and Cold and are commonly used for mild Exterior Wind-Cold syndrome. In regions with temperate climates, where Wind and Cold do not close the pores tightly, they are more often applied than Ma Huang and Gui Zhi for cold infections, influenza, certain stages of infectious childhood diseases and some skin diseases in which Exterior syndromes are involved. Meanwhile, they are also often used with pungent-cold herbs in syndromes where Wind-Heat is mixed with Wind-Cold. The patient may have symptoms such as chills, fever, thirst, sore throat and general pain. These two herbs are more often used in combination with cold herbs than Ma Huang and Gui Zhi.

Comparing Jing Jie with Fang Feng, Jing Jie is lighter and more dispersing. It is pungent but not strong, slightly warm but not dry. It is especially good at expelling Wind, no matter whether it is Wind-Cold or Wind-Heat. Moreover, it can expel Wind from the Blood so is often used in skin disorders when there is itching caused by Wind invasion, for instance in eczema, urticaria and food allergy. It is also used for infectious childhood diseases with Exterior syndrome and skin eruptions, such as measles, rubella, scarlet fever, chickenpox and so on.

Fang Feng is sweet, pungent and warm and enters the Bladder, Lung and Spleen meridians. As its sweet taste moderates the pungent taste, it is less strong in dispersing Wind on the surface of the body than Jing Jie. However, as it is warmer than Jing Jie and enters the Spleen meridian, it is especially good at expelling Dampness and Cold in the layers below the body surface, such as the subcutaneous region and muscles, which are controlled by the Spleen. When the patient feels pain and heaviness of the muscles, Fang Feng is more suitable than Jing Jie. This is also the reason that Fang Feng is more often used in Bi syndromes.

Although both herbs are gentle, they do have a pungent and warm nature, so both should be used with caution in patients without Wind invasion or in Yin deficiency with Empty-Heat.

DOWNWARD DRAINING HERBS

Downward Draining, or commonly known as Constipation is a condition of the digestive system, in which one cannot get rid of the unwanted residue of the foods and drinks consumed. Waste stays longer in the body and overtime starts to aggravate and enlarge intestinal pores, letting toxins enter the blood stream. Thus constipation is dangerous and should not be overlooked. The treatment principle for constipation is to drain the feces downward. In traditional Chinese medicine there are three types of downward draining herbs, that treat constipation – Purgatives, Moist Laxatives, and Harsh Expellants.

Purgatives treat constipation that manifests due to "internal heat", which dries out the fluids in the Large Intestine, making it difficult to expectorate the feces. "Internal cold" is another cause for accumulation, leading to weak peristalsis. It is also treated with purgatives (if you want to familiarize yourself with the concepts "internal heat" and "internal cold" visit the Physiology chapter of this project) In both cases purgative herbs respectively drain heat or warm the interior, and purge constipation.

Constipation can also develop because of internal dryness or Qi deficiency. Most commonly this is the case with elderly people as with aging the body's blood and energy level diminish, and the body's matter/substance (Yin) lessens. In these instances moist laxative herbs are used. They are gentle on the body yet have a lubricating effect on the intestines.

The third cause for constipation is accumulation of fluids, or poor water metabolism. In such cases the treatment principle is to induce diarrhea by using harsh expellants. Because these herbs strongly drive out excess water to clear accumulation they should be prescribed with care and only for short-term.

All purgatives and harsh expellants are contraindicated during pregnancy! Moist laxatives should be used with caution during pregnancy.

Major Chinese Herbs

A major purgative herb used in Chinese medicine is Da Huang (Rheum palmatum). Besides draining heat and purging accumulations this bitter, cold, yellow herb, translated as "big yellow", drains damp-heat and has antimicrobial effect. It also can be used for blood in the stool because of its property to drain heat from the blood, which manifests in bleeding.

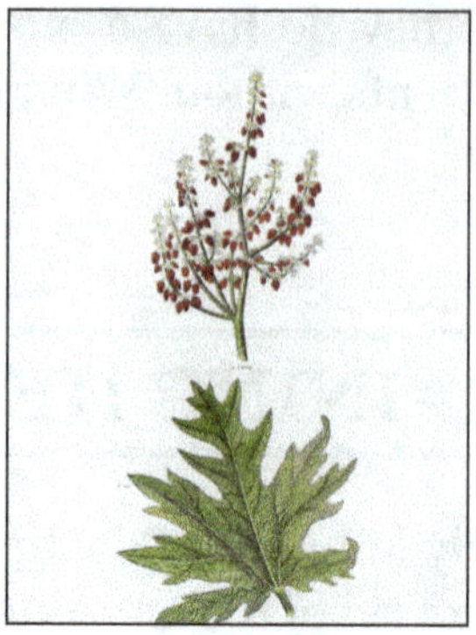

Another major purgative is Mang Xiao – mirabilite, also known as Glauber's salt. It purges accumulation and reduces redness and swelling in the eyes, mouth or throat due to heat.

Dried concentrate of the juice of aloe leaf – Lu Hui (Aloe Vera) –is gentle enough to be used for chronic constipation. It also kills parasites, especially roundworm.

Moist laxatives are Huo Ma Ren (Cannabis sativa) and Yu Li Ren (Prunus japonica). The first one is cannabis seeds. It moistens the intestines and nourishes Yin. The second herb is translated "constrained plum pit". It unblocks the bowels and reduces edema.

Morning glory is a beautiful deep-blue/purple flower, which seeds - Qian Niu Zi (P. purpurea) – are used as harsh expellants in Chinese medicine. They are helpful for water retention constipation, damp-heat accumulation constipation, food stagnation accumulation and parasites (roundworm and tapeworm). They also enter the Lung and benefit phlegm and congested fluids in the chest.

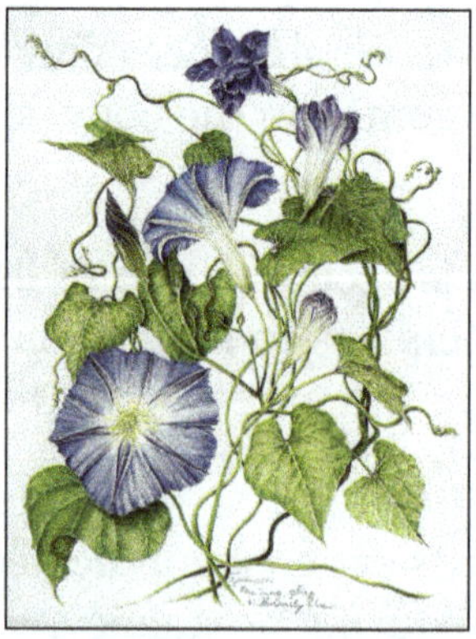

Yuan Hua (Daphne genkwa) is another flower with beautiful puprple color, that drains down water and is topically used to kill ringworm infestations. Gan Sui (Euphorbia kansui) is a violent harsh expellant root, which causes the water to pass anally. Ba Dou (Croton tiglium) – is a "hot" bean that is used for constipation due to accumulation of cold. It is also used for phlegm clogging the throat, causing difficulty breathing. Shang Lu (Phytolacca acinosa) is a root that benefits severe constipation and urinary difficulty.

CHINESE HERBS FOR PHLEGM-DAMPNESS

Phlegm-dampness is defined as chronic coughing with copious mucus that is white and thick in nature. Other symptoms include a stuffy feeling in the chest or gastric region, poor appetite, fatigue, and sometimes loose bowels. The tongue coating is white and greasy; the pulse is hesitant and rolling.

The remedy should invigorate the spleen, dry dampness, resolve phlegm and arrest coughing.

Sample prescription: Modified Citrus & Pinellia Decoction.

This is a classic formula for eliminating excessive phlegm and dampness, in which the pinellia tuber and poria work together to dry dampness and resolve phlegm; tangerine peel and liquorice root harmonize the spleen and promote its functioning. Additional herbs are necessary when particular symptoms are serious. For example:

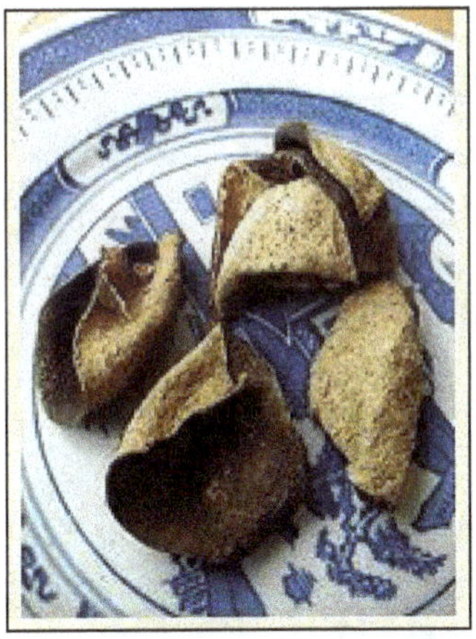

Dried tangerine peel.

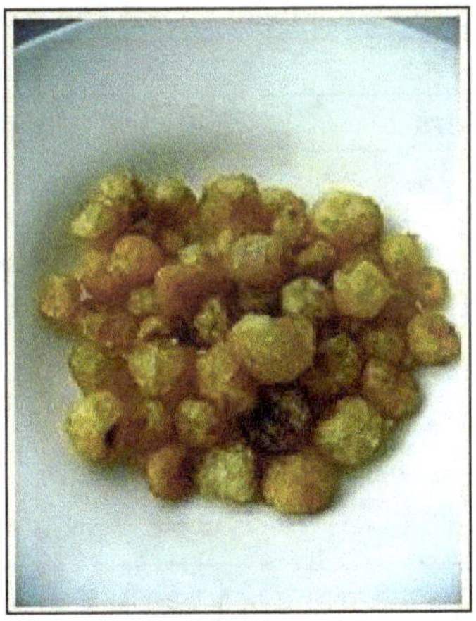

Pinellia tuber.

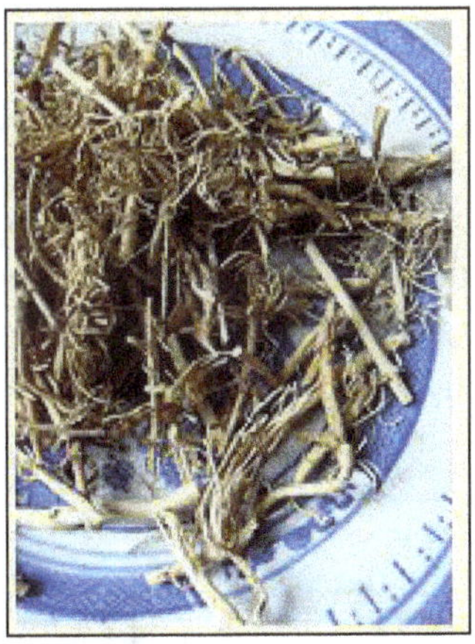

Cynanchum rhizome.

If individuals cough up profuse mucus and have stomach discomfort, the ability to eliminate the pathogens should further be enhanced with herbs like:

cang zhu	Atractylodes rhizome	Rhizoma Atractylodis
hou po	Magnolia bark	Cortex Magnoliae Officinalis
ku xing ren	Bitter apricot kernel	Semen Armeniacae Amarum
yi yi ren	Coix seed	Semen coicis

For severe coughing, the qi flows of lungs can be enhanced with herbs like:

ma huang	Ephedra	Herba Ephedrae
bai su zi	Perilla fruit	Fructus Perillae

ku xing ren	Bitter apricot kernel	Semen Armeniacae Amarum
bai qian	Cynanchum rhizome	Rhizoma Cynanchi Stauntonii

For severe fatigue and a pale tongue, select herbs to strengthen qi production of the spleen such as:

dang shen	Pilose asiabell root	Radix Codonopsis Pilosulae
bai shu	Largehead atractylodes rhizome	Rhizoma Atractylodis Macrocephalae

During the course of development, the accumulated pathogens can easily transform into heat or coldness evils, which further aggravates the cough or lead to other complex symptoms.

When mucus becomes thinner and the limbs are cold, the complexion is pale, a pale tongue with glossy coating, and a taut and slow pulse. The above prescription will be used together with Calm the Stomach Powder, so as to eliminate excessive dampness and coldness, otherwise, some warming herbs are selected:

xi xin	Manchurian wildginger	*Herba Asari*
gan jiang	fried ginger	*Rhizoma Zingiberis*
wu wei zi	schisandra	*Fructus Schisandrae*

When the mucus becomes thicker, difficult to expectorate or develops a fishy smell, and there is also a coarse breathing, thirst, a bitter taste in the mouth, and yellow greasy tongue coating, this indicates that a lung heat condition has developed. Clear Lung Heat and Resolve Phlegm Decoction will be more appropriate than the above prescription.

HERBAL REMEDIES FOR LIVER-FIRE TYPE

Liver-fire is frequent bouts of non-productive coughing, other accompanied symptoms include cough-induced chest pain, a flushed face, throat and mouth dryness. The symptoms usually fluctuate along with emotional changes. The tongue is red and covered by dry and yellow fur; the pulse is taut and rapid.

The remedy should clear the lungs, soothe the liver, smooth qi flow and check fire.

- Sample prescription: Modified Purging Lung Powder plus Indigo and Clam Shell Powder plus baical skullcap root.

In the prescription, the indigo and clam shell clear liver-heat and resolve phlegm; the baical skullcap root, mulberry root-bark and wolfberry root-bark clear the lung-heat; the rice and liquorice root nourish the stomach so as to replenish body fluids. Additional herbs are necessary when certain symptoms are obvious, for example:

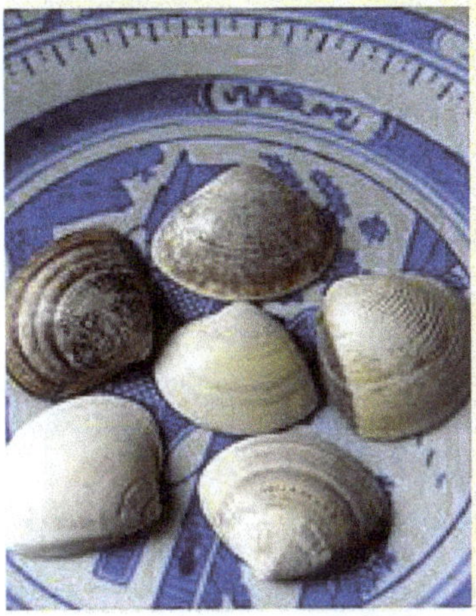

Clam shell.

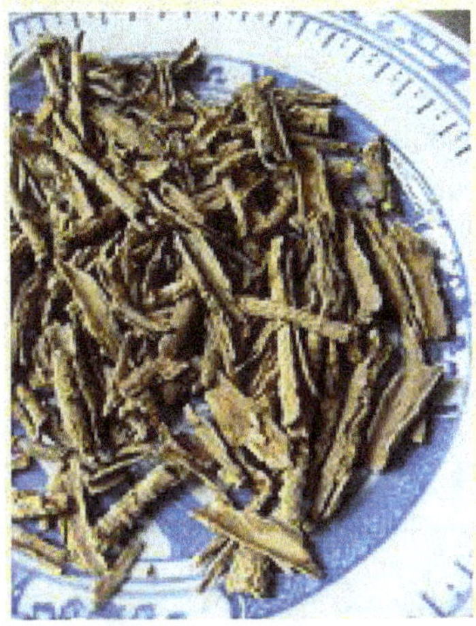

Wolfberry root-bark.

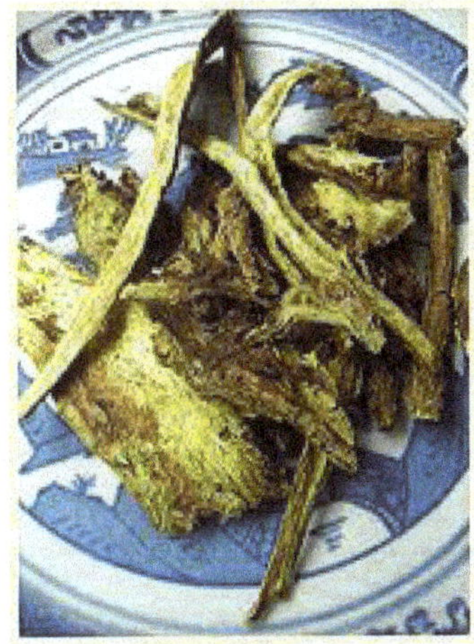

Baical skullcap root.

When there are symptoms like a flushed face and irritability, extra herbs are necessary to clear the liver-fire.

zhi zi	Gardenia fruit	Fructus Gardeniae
mu dan pi	Peony root bark	Crotex Moutan

Severe chest tightness and breath shortness can be relieved by smoothing lung qi with herbs like:

ting li zi	Pepperweed seed	Semen Lepidi
gua lou	Snakegourd peel	Fructus Trichosanthis
zhi ke	Bitter orange peel	Fructus Aurantii

TCM believes that chest or rib pain is a sign of stagnation in the liver meridian, and if this is the case other herbs should be added:

yu jin	Turmeric root-tuber	Radix Curcumae
si gua luo	Loofah	Retinervus Luffae Fructus

Excessive heat usually leads to sticky mucus which is difficult to expectorate; some herbs can help clear heat and promote expectoration:

hai fu shi	Pumice stone	
zhe bei	Thunberg fritillary bulb	Bulbus Fritillariae Thunbergii
dong gua ren	Winter gourd kernel	Semen Benincasae

Persistent coughing accompanied with excessive dryness in the throat and mouth, indicate that the lungs are damaged, and need proper nourishment. Suitable herbs include:

bei sha shen	Coastal glehnia root	Radix Glehniae
bai he	Lily bulb	Bulbus Lilii
mai dong	Dwarf lily-turf tuber	Radix Ophiopogonis
tian hua fen	Snakegourd root	Radix Trichosanthis
he zi	Myrobalan fruit	Fructus Chebulae

HERBAL REMEDIES FOR YIN DEFICIENCY

Yin deficiency is shown by a dry cough, or coughing up blood. Other symptoms include hot flushes in the afternoon, red cheeks, warm palms and soles, insomnia, night sweats, fatigue and irritability. The tongue is red, and the pulse is thready and rapid.

The remedy should nourish the lungs, clear lung-heat, resolve phlegm and arrest coughing.

- Sample prescription: Modified glehnia root and dwarf lily-turf tuber decoction.

In the prescription, the glehnia root, Solomonseal rhizome, dwarf lily-turf tuber and snakegourd root nourish the lungs and promote the production of body fluids; the mulberry leaf dispels heat and dryness evils through the body surface; the liquorice root and hyacinth bean reinforce the spleen to produce more nutrient essence, so as to support lung functioning. Additional herbs are necessary when particular symptoms are obvious, for example:

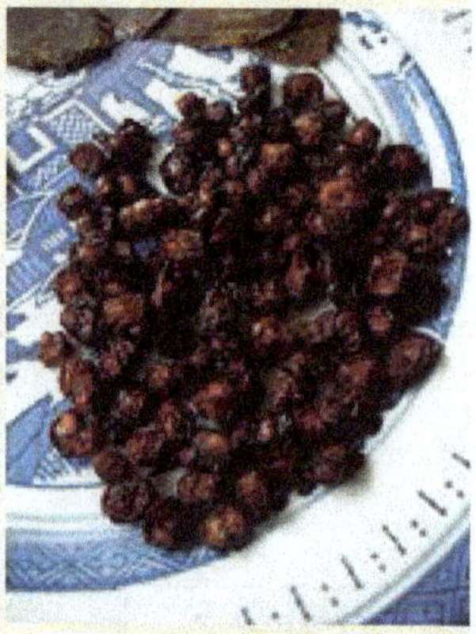

Schisandra.

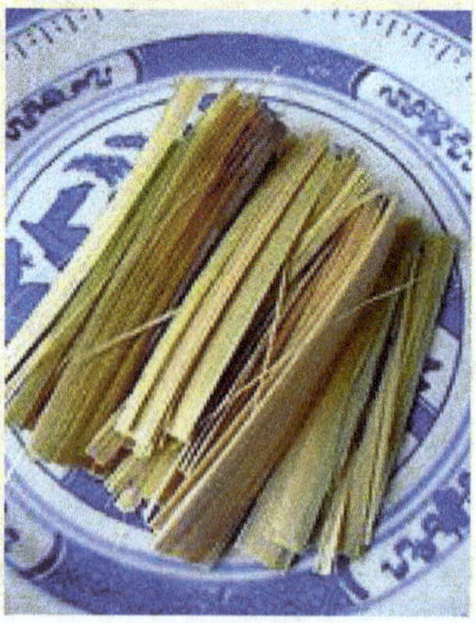

Bamboo shavings.

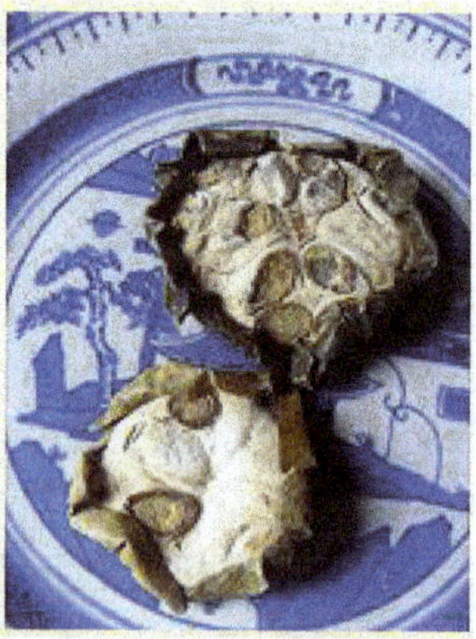

Snakegourd peel.

In case if the cough has persisted for a long time, the lungs must have accumulated a lot of heat, therefore, more heat-clearing herbs are necessary. In the prescription, delete the mulberry leaf, and add:

sang bai pi	White mulberry root-bark	Cortex Mori Radicis
di gu pi	Wolfberry root-bark	Lycii Radicis Cortex

Severe cough may need extra force to calm the lung qi, so add herbs like:

chuan bei mu	Unibract fritillary bulb	Bulbus Fritillariae Cirrhosae
ku xing ren	Bitter apricot kernel	Semen Armeniacae Amarum
bai bu	Stemona root	Radix stemonae

Coughing accompanied with breath shortness indicates that lung qi should be reconsolidated with the following herbs:

wu wei zi	Schisandra	Fructus Schisandrae
he zi	Myrobalan fruit	Fructus Chebulae

Coughing up yellow and thick mucus indicates that the lungs has generated their own heat, more herbs should be added to clear heat and resolve phlegm:

ha ke	Clam shell	Concha Meretricis Seu Cyclinae
zhi mu	Anemarrhena rhizome	Rhizoma Anemarrhenae
gua lou	Snakegourd pccl	Fructus Trichosanthis
zhu ru	Bamboo shavings	Caulis Bambusae in Taeniam
huang qin	Baical skullcap root	Radix Scutellariae

Coughing up blood, indicate that the blood is over-heated, suitable cooling herbs are:

zhi zi	Gardenia fruit	Fructus Gardeniae
mu dan pi	Peony root-bark	Crotex Moutan
bai mao gen	Couch grass rhizome	Rhizoma Imperatae
bai ji	Common bletilla tuber	Rhizoma Bletillae
ou jie	Lotus rhizome-node	Nodus Nelumbinis Rhizomatis

Severe hot flashes or low-grade fever can be arrested by:

yin chai hu	Starwort root	Radix Stellariae
qing hao	Sweet wormwood herb	Herba artemisiae Annuae
bai wei	Blackened swallowwort root	Radix Cynanchi Atrati

Excessive night sweats can be arrested by:

nuo dao gen	Root of glutinous rice straw	Radis Ophiopogan
fu xiao mai	Shriveled wheat	Fructus Tritici Levis

When coughing is accompanied with wheezing or breathing difficulties, kidney qi deficiency may also appear, and the depleted state can be reconsolidated with herbs like:

shu di	Processed rhemannia rhizome	Rhizoma Rehmanniae Praeparatae
shan zhu yu	Cornus fruit	Fructus Corni
wu wei zi	Schisandra	Fructus Schisandrae
ren shen	Ginseng	Radix Ginseng
ge jie	Tokay	Gekko

CHINESE EXTERNAL HERBAL REMEDIES FOR INSOMNIA

In traditional Chinese medicine (TCM) theory, our body consists of a giant web called the meridian system that distributes the fundamental substances over the body. Along the channels, acupoints are the sites where the qi of the organs and meridians infuse onto the body surface, and simulating these points help regulate the corresponding organs or meridians and promote the recovery of internal disharmonies.

To treat insomnia, regardless of cause, the basic principle is to resume harmony between the body and mind, so that a natural rhythm of sleep and waking can return. An external herbal remedy is an effective and easy way to relax and induce sleep. The selected herbs are made into a paste, powder, solution, medicinal wine or essential oil. The active components of the preparations are absorbed through the skin or acupoints and transmitted by the meridian system to finally work on the target organs.

Herbal Pillows and Sachets to Promote Sleep

Appropriate bedding promotes a restful night and ensures that the body maintains a healthy vitality. Herbal stuffing used to make pillows and sachets are natural sedatives, as the selected herbs are mostly aromatic and are able to remove blockages, calming and relieving the stress in the body.

Prescription

Chrysanthemum (100g), magnetite (100g), albizia flower (100g), tuber fleeceflower stem (100g), common rush (30g), clove (30g), acorus (60g), polygala root (60g), Indian bread with pine (60g), sandal wood (10g) and borneol (10g). When seriously disturbed by dreams, add fossil bone (100g) and oyster shell (60g). Grind the ingredients properly.

Bamboo shavings, chrysanthemum, mulberry leaf, peppermint, oriental arborvitae leafy-twig, Dahurian angelica root, Sichuan lovage, schizonepeta herb, peony root bark and magnetite. Mix equal amounts of each ingredient and crush them slightly.

Peppermint, chrysanthemum, lophatherum herb, sweet wormwood herb, fortune eupatorium herb and tuber fleeceflower stem, 30g of each; fossil bone, oyster shell, and ochre minerals, 30g for each; Sichuan lovage, Dahurian angelica root, Chinese nardostachyos root, vitex fruit, costustoot, silkworm dung, tangerine peel and atractylodes rhizome, 10g each; Manchurian wildginger, acorus, Chinese honeylocust abnormal fruit and borneol, 5g each. Mix and grind properly.

Mix all the ingredients together, place in a cloth bag and sew up the end, tuck inside a pillow or cushion to give off a gentle fragrance during the day or while sleeping. These mixtures need renewing after several months. The room temperature should be around 25-30 °C.

Age, body type, specific health problem, and even season of the year should be considered when selecting herbs.

Considerations	Suitable ingredients
Yin deficiency with virtual fire	Mung bean, black soybean
Yang hyperactive	Selfheal fruit spike, silkworm dung
Ear ringing or poor hearing	Magnetite
Blurred or poor vision	Chrysanthemum, tea leaf and cassia seed
Nervous debility or heart problems	Amber, Chinese arborvitae kernel
Hot summer	Bamboo shavings, gypsum

Topical Herbal Dressings to Promote Sleep

The prescribed herbs are ground or extracted, made into a paste and applied to areas like the navel, soles or palms to induce sleep. By stimulating the specific acupoints of the various regions, a medicinal effect infiltrates the skin and reaches the meridians, activating qi movement and promoting internal balance.

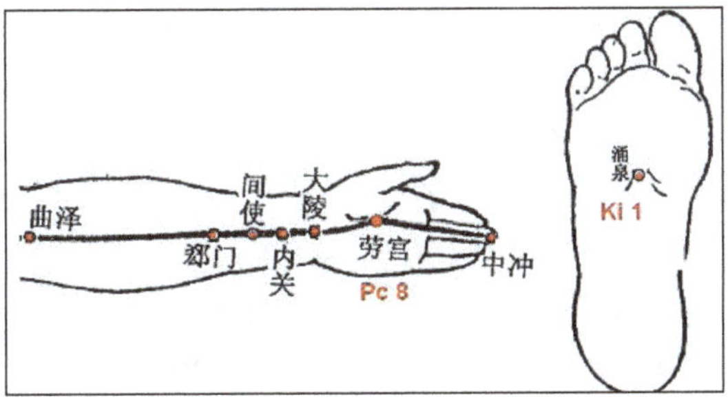

Important body points for TCM external herbal remedies.

Dressing for the palms:

Prescription: fossil bone (20g), amber (5g), pearl (4.5g), golden thread rhizome (5g) and pinellia tuber (10g). Grind into a fine powder and put aside. Every night before going to bed, take 3-4g of the powder and mix with an oral solution called Fresh Bamboo Juice (xian zhu li ye) or just tap water, paste on the centre of both palms, cover with swabs and fixed in place. Afterward, press with fingers on the area for 30 minutes each, keeping the dressing overnight. Apply for 20 days as one course. In the centre of the palm, an acupoint called lao gong (Pc 8) belongs to the pericardium meridian, it works with the ingredients to calm the spirit and promote sleep.

Dressing for the umbilicus:

Prescription: Red sage root (20g), sulfur (20g), polygala root (20g) and acorus (20g). Acorus (10g), turmeric (10g), immature bitter orange (10g), Chinese eaglewood (10g), sour jujube seed (10g) and amber (10g). Medicinal evodia fruits (100g).

Grind the above ingredients into a fine powder and put aside. Every night before going to bed, take 5g of the powder and mix with a small amount of rice wine into paste form, fill in the navel (or umbilicus) and then cover by gauze or tape. The umbilicus is known as shen que (Cv 8), which is an important acupoint along the conception vessel, works with the ingredients to calm the spirit and induce sleep.

Dressing for the soles:

Prescription: Arisaema with bile (10g), Sichuan lovage (30g), golden thread rhizome (20g). Golden thread rhizome (30g) and Cassia bark (30g).

Grind the ingredients into a powder and put aside. Every night before going to bed, mix 5g of the powder with honey, paste it on the soles of the feet, and then cover by gauze or tape. There is an acupoint named yong quan (Ki 1) in the cent re of the soles, which is an important point along the kidney meridian. It works with the ingredients to promote communication between heart and kidney, and calms the mind.

Wet dressing on the forehead:

Prescription: Magnetite (20g), Indian bread with pine (15g), schisandra (10g) and prickly acanthopanax root (20g). Boil the magnetite with 1500 ml of water for 30 minutes, then add in other ingredients, boil for 30 minutes and filter out the solution. Pinellia tuber (12g), poria (9g), tangerine peel (9g), arisaema with bile (9g), acorus (9g), polygala root (9g), lophatherum herb (9g), immature bitter orange (6g), liquorice root (6g, processed with honey). Boil the ingredients with 1000ml of water for 30 minutes and filter out the solution.

Every night when in bed, soak the gauze in the warm solution and use it to cover on the forehead and eyes. This method stimulates and harmonizes the meridians and soothes the mind.

Herbal Foot Baths to Promote Sleep

The feet are the end of three yang meridians (stomach, gall bladder, bladder), and the start of three yin meridians (spleen, liver, kidney). There are more than sixty acupoints located on each foot, and appropriate stimulation on them can activate the flows in the meridians, and enhance body functioning. In modern understanding, soaking the feet dilates the local blood vessels, induces blood flow downward, which relieves the congested state of the brain and relaxes the mind to prepare for sleep. Foot-soaking remedies are not only for relieving foot strain, but is also a simple and effective way to promote health.

Insomnia prescription for foot bathing:

Prescription: Magnetite (50g), sore jujube seed (30g), Chinese arborvitae kernel (30g), tuber fleeceflower stem (15g) and angelica root (20g). Magnetite (50g), chrysanthemum (15g), baical skullcap root (15g) and tuber fleeceflower stem (15g).

Boil the above ingredients, and soak the feet for 20 minutes in the solution every night before sleep. The ingredients help calm the spirit and promote a restful sleep.

Insomnia accompanied by irritability:

Prescription: gambir vine stem (20g) and borneol (3g). Crush the gambir vine stem, place the ingredients in a gauze bag and put in a basin with hot water. Stir slightly to let the active ingredients release properly. When the water becomes warm, insert the feet and soak for 15 minutes. Soak twice a day, in the morning and before sleep.

Insomnia accompanied by hypertension:

Prescription: Magnetite (30g), abalone shell (30g), astragalus root (20g), angelica root (20g), cassia twig (20g), eucommia bark (20g) and caltrop fruit (20g). Crush magnetite and abalone shell properly and boil with 3000ml of water for 30 minutes, then add the other ingredients and boil for another 30 minutes more before filtering the solution. Pour the solution into a basin, cool down for a while and soak the feet in it for 30 minutes, keep the solution at 40-50 °C while soaking.

Insomnia due to mental fatigue:

Prescription: Polygala root (20g), golden thread rhizome (10g), poria (20g), acorus (20g) and pilose asiabell root (20g). Place the ingredients in a gauze bag and then place in a basin with hot water; when the water turns warm, insert the feet and soak for 30 minutes.

Sleep disturbed by dreams and early awakening:

Prescription: Frankincense (15g), sour jujube seed (30g), angelica root (30g), fossil bone (50g), schisandra (10g), rehmannia root (50g) and red sage root (50g). Boil the above ingredients, and soak the feet in the solution for 30 minutes.

For individuals who prefer a whole body treatment, they can also enjoy herbal baths, saunas or steam methods. The heat of the water helps release the properties of the herbs, and also opens the skin pores, which facilitate the herbs being absorbed through the skin and so into the bloodstream, benefiting both the mind and body.

HERBS FOR SHEN DISORDERS

The way Chinese herbs are used for shen disorders has changed over time and is affected by cultural differences among the countries utilizing Chinese medicine. For example, the three syndromes describe in the previous chapter (and the contribution of "hidden water" or "water toxin") have been of interest in ancient times in China and in Japan today, but herb formulas presented in modern Chinese texts often have yet a different focal point.

Further, the selection of ingredients to use in treatments has changed, especially in recent years, and particularly as one takes the formulas from Asia and tries to utilize them in Western countries, where there are different concepts of what serves as an acceptable ingredient. For example, the most revered of the ingredients for shen disorders (and for several other conditions) in China throughout the past 2,000 years is one which we no longer would even consider using, but its ancient description is worth relaying:

> Dansha is sweet and slightly cold. It treats hundreds of diseases of the five viscera and the body. It nurtures the essence spirit (jingshen), quiets the hun and po, boosts the qi brightens the eyes, and kills spirit demons and evil ghosts. Protracted taking may enable one to communicate with the spirit light and prevent senilit.

This compound, cinnabar, was one of many mineral agents that were relied upon for such spiritual aims. It is a mercury compound that the Chinese believed was safe to use, and which had been used routinely until just a few years ago. The stories about "contaminated" Chinese herb products that are relayed in Western countries often reflected detection of mercury from cinnabar, as well as arsenic from realgar, two items that had been trusted by the physicians in China. This was not contamination, but intentional inclusion of the ingredients.

Animal parts were also used for the spirit remedies, including this one that we also don't use today:

> Shexiang is acrid and warm. It mainly keeps off malignant qi, kills ghosts and [adverse] spiritual matters, [cures] malaria, gu toxins [certain types of parasites], epilepsy, and tetany, and removes the three worms. Protracted taking may eliminate evils to prevent depressive ghost dreams in sleep.

This substance, musk, is from an endangered deer species mainly found in the mountainous area of Tibet and adjacent mountainous Chinese provinces, and was commonly employed in remedies for reviving consciousness because of its potent fragrance. Endangered species concerns have eliminated from use numerous animal substances that were considered of great value. Further, European governments have somewhat arbitrarily restricted virtually all animal ingredients from use in "herbal" formulas.

A mineralized animal substance, dragon bone (fossilized bones of large mammals, so no animal material remains), was long employed as a spirit medicine:

> Longgu is sweet and balanced. It mainly treats heart and abdominal demonic influx, [adverse] spiritual matters, old ghosts, cough, and counterflow [of qi], diarrhea and dysentery of pus and blood.

Dragon bone is still in use; dragon teeth is collected from similar source materials and used similarly (though especially for treatment of disorders associated with fright). Fossilized tree resins, in the form of amber (also called succinum; the Chinese name is hupo, referring to the po soul of the tiger, which it is said to represent), are included in traditional and modern formulas for spirit disorders.

Ordinary plant materials are the main ingredients in spirit formulations, and the best known of these is ginseng. Due to attempts to vigorously promote its sale in the West, the applications of this herb have been altered to serving primarily as an energy tonic, a use quite different than in traditional Chinese medicine:

> Renshen is sweet and a little cold. It mainly supplements the five viscera. It quiets the essence spirit [jingshen], settles the hun and po, checks fright palpitations, eliminates evil qi, brightens the eyes, opens the heart, and sharpens the wits.

The case of ginseng is an example of how information about herb use can become distorted. As a result, many people worry that ginseng will have an agitating quality when, in fact, it is used in the Chinese formulas as a calming substance.

There are some principles of therapy that have changed due to the developments of modern medicine. For example, throughout the history of Chinese medicine several shen disturbances, including loss of consciousness, mania, and emotional agitation, were understood to occur as the direct result of feverish diseases. Thus, herbs that purge fire, including rhino horn (no longer used), raw rehmannia (sheng dihuang), coptis (huanglian), gardenia (shanzhizi), moutan (mudanpi), and scute (huangqin), were sometimes key ingredients in the prescriptions. In modern times, most of these feverish conditions can be controlled with antibiotics, antipyretic drugs, and other modern therapies (or can be prevented outright by vaccination) so that the mind and brain disorders that are the subject of potential Chinese-herbal treatment today are rarely associated with febrile disease. While these same fire-purging herbs have some sedative effects, it is clear from the ancient formula descriptions that they were included mainly for their role in treating a febrile condition.

As a result of research done during the 20th Century, modern Chinese practitioners have turned much of their attention to the principle of treating blood stasis, which was less frequently described in ancient times. While xue dao zheng usually involved the problem of abdominal stagnation of blood flow, today's efforts are usually directed at blood stasis affecting the heart and brain, looking particularly at the problem of strokes and other diseases of aging associated with vascular blockage. Ingredients such as red peony (chishao), cnidium (chuanxiong), persica (taoren), carthamus (honghua), and salvia (danshen) are the most frequently relied upon for these purposes.

Thus, one can say that some principles of therapy now have less emphasis than before (i.e., clearing heat) and others have more emphasis than before (i.e., vitalizing blood), and this is important to recognize when analyzing formulas described in modern clinical reports from China. Similarly, some ingredients are less often used, such as animal substances, while others are more frequently used, especially those plant materials that have escaped worries about toxicity and endangered species status.

Basic Therapeutic Approaches

There are four main therapeutic approaches using herbs in traditional Chinese medicine to address the problems classified as spirit disorders:

Tonification therapy: The brain is described as an extension of the marrow which belongs to the kidney system, so herbs that nourish the kidney are understood to nourish the brain (and spinal cord). Lack of nourishment (particularly of the fluid component, that is, yin and blood) of any organ can lead to mental distress, due to the fact that the internal spirits cannot rest if their associated internal organs are "empty," that is, deficient in essential fluids. In particular, deficiency of liver and heart can easily cause disturbance of the mind (due to hyperactivity of the hun and shen). Weakness of spleen qi is often ultimately responsible for lack of nourishment of all the organs and the body; the spleen also promotes upward circulation of qi to reach the brain.

Regulating qi: The free flow of visceral qi, regulated by the liver, is understood to correspond to the mental condition, particularly the thought processes and the reactions to experiences. For example, stagnated (depressed) liver qi circulation corresponds to mental depression, repetitive thoughts, limited outlook, and other mental conditions that, in turn, cause problems in social situations, furthering the liver qi stagnation. Although anger is the emotion frequently cited as associated with the liver and its circulation of qi, in fact, other emotions also have various effects on the qi, and the consequence may be stagnation of liver qi circulation.

Calming agitation: Aside from the problem of deficiency that leads to unsettling of the spirit, the mind can be agitated as a result of heat, wind, or uprushing qi and yang, disorders that may be secondary to deficiency (e.g., yin deficiency of the liver yields liver fire and internal wind) or may be an excess pattern (from a pathogenic influence or from diet, excess emotions, etc.). Herbs are used to clear the heat (purge fire), sedate the wind, and settle the upward rising of qi and yang.

Clearing orifices of phlegm-mist: The connection between the heart and mind (or brain) is made by channels (orifices) that can become obstructed; the ultimate source of the obstruction may be weak stomach/spleen function leading to accumulation of phlegm, or fire syndrome damaging fluids and transforming them to pathological phlegm. Aromatic and penetrating herbs can clear the obstruction and phlegm-resolving herbs can help prevent the orifices from becoming obstructed again.

In designing a formulation, it is common to rely primarily on one or more of the first three methods listed here to treat shen disorders. In fact, tonification therapy is a part of nearly all the treatments used in modern practice. The fourth method (which will be analyzed more fully in the appendix to this chapter), is especially used in cases of severe disturbance, for ailments associated with the phlegm syndrome, and for treatment of elderly patients.

Tables some sample herbs in each of the four therapeutic areas of primary concern. The herbs were selected for inclusion in these tables on the basis of high frequency of use in treating mind and brain disorders as described in both the traditional and modern literature (the formulas for treating the disorders will be described in the next two chapters). Some items frequently mentioned in traditional literature (e.g., musk, rhino horn, cinnabar) and used until recently in China have been retained here to assist in the study of that literature.

Within each category, the herbs are listed alphabetically by common name (followed by pinyin and typical botanical source for clear identification). In the section of "main actions," the information is derived primarily from Oriental Materia Medica (2), with only those actions that are relevant to treatment of mental disorders included in the table. Since the concept of phlegm-mist is not often elucidated, an extensive explanation is presented in the appendix.

Table: Tonic therapies frequently used for shen disorders.

Herb	Main Actions	Comments
Alpinia*yizhiren Alpinia oxyphylla*	Supplements spleen, warms the kidney, astringes essence, fortifies qi	The Chinese name means to enhance the disposition of the individual (increase wisdom, is one translation). It is thought to improve the thinking function associated with the spleen and the will associated with the kidney.
Asparagus*tianmendong Asparagus cochinchinensis*	Nourishes yin, moistens dryness	Asparagus is considered similar in nature, taste, and function to ophiopogon and is commonly used in combination with it to nourish the yin.

Astragalus*huangqi* *Astragalus membrana-ceous*	Supplements qi, increases yang	Astragalus helps the spleen generate a pure and clear qi that rises upward to nourish the heart and brain
Atractylodes*baizhu* *Atractylodes macro-cephalla*	Supplements spleen, tonifies qi	This aromatic tonic for the spleen disperses stagnated fluids that can obscure the heart orifices.
Cistanche*roucongrong* *Cistanche salsa*	Nourishes kidney essence, supplements yang	The soft, black, salty herb is thought to quickly nourish the deficient kidney essence, invigorating yang without harming the yin.
Codonopsis*dangshen* *Codonopsis pilosula*	Invigorates the spleen and stomach, replenishes qi	In China, codonopsis is almost always used as a substitute for ginseng as a stomach/spleen tonic, but it lacks the spirit-calming qualities of ginseng.
Cornus*wuzhuyu* *Cornus officinalis*	Supplements liver and kidney, astringes essence	The sour fruit is frequently used to astringe and nourish the essence and help prevent deterioration of health.
Cuscuta*tusizi* *Cuscuta chinensis*	Supplements kidney essence, clears vision	The seed is thought to help prevent leakage of essence (as an astringent), therefore it is used to prevent deterioration. It gently tonifies yang, without harming yin.
Dioscorea*shanyao* *Dio-scorea batatas*	Supplements spleen, stomach and kidneys, astringes essence	Dioscorea is used in many treatments for weakening of the kidney essence; its ability to benefit the spleen at the same time is unusual among the Chinese herbs for that purpose.
Ginseng*renshen* *Panax ginseng*	Replenishes and supplements original qi, benefits the five viscera, pacifies the spirit, soothes the soul, increases wisdom	Ginseng is one of the original remedies for spirit disorders used in Chinese medicine; it has a calming nature and replenishes all deficiencies. In the West, ginseng has taken on the connotation of an energy stimulant; practitioners and patients often worry about the proclaimed stimulant action of this herb.
Ho-shou-wu*heshouwu* *Polygonum multiflorum*	Nourishes yin, replenishes essence and blood, tonifies liver and kidneys	Ho-shou-wu is a famous "anti-aging" herb that is reputed to keep the body and mind young and active. By nourishing the kidney and liver, it nourishes the brain.
Hoelen*fuling* *Poria cocos*	Strengthens spleen, harmonizes middle warmer, tranquilizes the heart, pacifies the spirit, resolves moisture	Hoelen is used to soak up excess moisture and improve spleen function; it is also favored as a sedative. It has a mild action. The sedative fu-shen is from the same source.
Longan*longyanroux* *Euphoria longana*	Supplements the heart, stabilizes the spirit, tonifies spleen, nourishes blood	This sedative tonic has properties that imitate the actions of ginseng plus tang-kuei. It is primarily used in Ginseng and Longan Combination (*Guipi Tang*).
Lycium*gouqizi* *Lycium barbarum*	Supplements liver and kidneys, promotes production of essence and blood	Lycium is commonly used in cases of essence deficiency and is considered especially useful because of its mild nature, not producing any adverse digestive effects even in large dosage.

Ophiopogon*maimendong* *Ophiopogon japonicus*	Nourishes yin, moistens dryness, removes heat, resolves phlegm, calms spirit	This yin-nourishing herb is especially relied upon when there is phlegm accumulation and heart agitation; sometimes asparagus is added to enhance the heat clearing action.
Peony *baishao* *Paeonia alba*	Supplements blood, vitalizes blood, cools blood, astringes liver yin, strengthens spleen	Peony is the most commonly used blood nourishing herb because its other properties (vitalizing and cooling blood, astringing liver yin) take care of several requirements of the formulations.
Rehmannia *shudihuang* *Rehmannia glutinosa*	Nourishes blood, yin, and essence, supplements kidney and liver	This rich, black processed root is considered one of the most important herbs to nourish the liver and kidney. It is used to prevent and even reverse the deterioration associated with aging.
Tang-kuei *danggui* *Angelica sinensis*	Supplements and moves blood	This herb is used for nourishing the blood of the liver and heart, which has the effects of controlling emotional distress and relieving spasms.

Table: Qi-regulating Herbs. Bupleurum is included in this table as an important qi regulating herb, particularly for shen disorders, but in the Materia Medica it is placed in the surface relieving category, which reflected one of its most frequent uses at the time the herb categories were established; magnolia bark is categorized with aromatic moisture resolving herbs, but it has an important role in regulating qi circulation and so is included here.

Herb	Main Actions	Comments
Bupleurum *chaihu* *Bupleurum chinense*	Regulates liver qi, raises yang qi	Bupleurum strongly dredges liver qi; this action may be uncomfortable in those with blood deficiency (it is often administered with blood tonics); it also aids rising of qi, so that herbs to lower qi may be needed in the formula.
Chih-ko *zhiqiao* *Citrus aurantium*	Disperses central qi, regulates horizontal qi circulation; resolves phlegm	Used for food stagnancy, epigastric aching, and lung congestion; it is often used to aid bupleurum in dispersing qi and to aid pinellia in resolving phlegm.
Chih-shih *zhishi Citrus aura tium* (unripe fruit)	Disperses central qi, regulates vertical qi circulation; purges gallbladder, clears heat and phlegm	Used for abdominal stagnation with constipation; helps direct qi flow downward. Chih-shih is helpful in reducing damp-heat and phlegm accumulation especially that associated with gallbladder stagnation or heat.
Citrus *chenpi Citrus reticulata*	Disperses qi, strengthens spleen, dries moisture and phlegm	The most widely used qi-regulating herb; it is also used in treatment of most phlegm disorders, combined with pinellia. Citrus aids the spleen in dispersing moisture.
Cyperus *xiangfu, xiangfuzi* *Cyperus rotundus*	Strongly disperses central qi, alleviates pain, regulates menstruation	Analgesic for headaches and abdominal pains and alleviates qi stagnation; this is considered an important herb for treating depression.

Lindera *wuyao Lindera strychnifolia*	Disperses qi alleviates pain, warms the kidney	This herb is used like bupleurum to disperse stagnant qi, but is especially used in cold syndromes and for weak kidney qi.
Magnolia bark *houpu Magnolia obovata*	Dries dampness, moves qi	Mainly used for abdominal distention, up-rushing of qi, food stagnation, obstruction of phlegm, and tightness of the diaphragm.
Saussurea *muxiang Saussurea lappa* or *Jrinea soulei*	Disperses qi, alleviates pain, controls diarrhea, sedative	Used for mainly for abdominal disorders that include diarrhea.

Table: Sedative Herbs. Polygala, listed in the Materia Medica among the heart-nourishing herbs, has been listed both here and in the category of herbs to help resolve phlegm mist.

Herb	Main Actions	Comments
Biota *baiziren* *Biota orientalis*	Nourishes heart and calms mind	This seed is very oily, so it is used only in moderate dosage if there is a spleen-damp syndrome, but is favored for constipation and dryness.
Cinnabar *zhusha* mercuric sulfide	Sedates the heart and calms the mind	This is the premier sedative of the Chinese tradition and mentioned in numerous ancient and modern formulas; however, it is avoided in the West due to its content of mercury, the active constituent.
Dragon bone *longgu* fossil bones	Pacifies the liver, restrains floating yang, sedates and calms the mind	These are fossilized bones of ice age animals, comprised mainly of soluble minerals, such as calcium carbonate. It has a nutritive and calming action. It is also an astringent for kidney essence.
Dragon teeth *longchi* fossil teeth	Sedates and calms the spirit	Like dragon bones, dragon teeth are fossilized; Chinese doctors regard them as especially useful for fright-induced mental disorders.
Fu-shen *fushen* *Poria cocos + Pinus sp.*	Sedative, moisture-resolving, strengthens spleen	Fu-shen is mostly the same material as hoelen with similar properties, but includes portions of pine root; the pine confers a sedative effect.
Oyster shell *muli* *Ostrea gigas*	Pacifies the liver and restrains the floating yang	Oyster shell is used to calm agitation; it has astringent properties and also reduces excess stomach acid. It mainly contains calcium carbonate.
Polygala *yuanzhi* *Polygala tenuifolia*	Stabilizes the heart, calms the mind, disperses phlegm	Polygala is a nourishing sedative, often combined with zizyphus; it is commonly used with acorus to disperse phlegm-mist and enliven the mental functions.
Schizandra *wuweizi* *Schizandra chinensis*	Astringes essence, calms agitation	Like cornus, it is relied upon to astringe essence and prevent deterioration of health; modern research has shown that it normalizes cerebral electrical discharges and is thus used in treatments for brain disorders, especially for insomnia and poor memory.

Succinum *hupo* fossilized resin	Sedates and calms spirit, vitalizes blood circulation	This is the aged resin mostly from various pine trees; the ancient Chinese said that this material is actually the soul of tigers that have died, and it has a sedating quality that still imparts the tiger's power.
Zizyphus *suanzaoren Zizyphus spinosa*	Nourishes heart and calms spirit, nourishes liver	The most commonly-used sedative especially treats mental disorders characterized by insomnia and agitation.

What is Phlegm-Mist affecting the Orifices of the Heart?

Before presenting the herbs for phlegm-mist, the nature of this condition is first described. Although phlegm-mist can affect different parts of the body, the terminology of "phlegm misting the orifices of the heart" (tanmi xinqiao) is frequently used for the concept as it refers to function of the brain and the syndrome that produces or worsens shen disorders.

The condition is sometimes described as phlegm entering the heart, or as phlegm entering the heart meridian (or "channel"). The original description of meridians in the Chinese medical system is related to blood vessels. We know this, in part, because virtually all mentions of the flow of qi in the ancient texts are actually about the combined flow of "qi and blood." It is easy to become confused about the Chinese view of human physiology when modern writers describe meridians as pathways existing solely for the flow of qi, to be distinguished from blood vessels for the flow of blood, which is not consistent with the prior 2,000 years of Chinese literature. The fact that the meridian maps (for acupuncture) do not correspond with blood vessels merely indicates that what was eventually mapped for purposes of describing acupuncture therapies failed to follow precisely the underlying traditional conceptual framework. When describing long-held ideas about human physiology such as this, it is important to consider the context, and in this case, the flow of qi and blood were considered to be unified and involved the same "vessels."

Phlegm mist is a concept that can be traced back at least to the Song Dynasty. By that time, Chinese doctors were distinguishing "substantial" phlegm (such as sputum, which is described as "condensed pathological fluid") and "insubstantial phlegm" or "hidden phlegm" (such as the mist of the heart orifices; a "thin pathological fluid"). The substantial phlegm would mainly accumulate in the lungs and stomach and could be noted in the sinuses and throat, while the insubstantial phlegm would accumulate in the meridians, distributing to various parts of the body, such as the heart orifices and the brain (e.g., causing dizziness or loss of consciousness in severe cases), the lymph nodes (causing nodules and swellings), and the limbs (e.g., causing numbness). The two types of phlegm were thought to have the same origin and the same fundamental nature, but would permeate different parts of the body (the thick sputum could not penetrate the meridians, but the insubstantial phlegm could).

Further, insubstantial phlegm can combine with other pathological influences to yield phlegm-fire, wind-phlegm, and phlegm-turbidity. According to the doctrine that evolved, the phlegm mist when combined with the other pathological factors-such as fire, wind, or damp-could produce more severe symptoms. Its material nature would capture the more ethereal forces of fire or wind to make the disease persist; similarly, the phlegm mist could blend with damp to yield turbidity that obscures the clear flow of qi and yang to the brain, interfering with normal mental and sensory functions, though not completely blocking the circulation to the brain except in the worst cases, in which case one might suffer what we understand today to be a stroke.

Diseases and symptoms attributed to phlegm mist affecting the heart orifices in addition to stroke paralysis affecting the major muscles (hemiplegia), include dizziness, loss of consciousness (coma), mania (emotional outbursts, disturbed speech), convulsions (especially epilepsy), sudden sensory loss (deafness, blurred vision, loss of taste and smell, inability to speak), lockjaw, and stiff tongue. Several of these symptoms may be the result of strokes. Diseases currently treated in China by herbs that resolve phlegm-mist affecting the heart orifices also include manic-depressive disorder and senile dementia (Alzheimer's disease).

Table: Herbs that Clear Phlegm Mist and Open the Orifices. In addition to herbs in the Materia Medica categories of opening orifices and resolving phlegm, this table includes curcuma, a blood vitalizing herb with phlegm-resolving action. Silkworm, a wind-calming herb, and polygala, a heart-nourishing sedative, both also help resolve phlegm mist, so are included here.

Herb	Main Actions	Comments
Acorus *changpu* *Acorus gramineus*	Opens orifices, expels phlegm and turbidity, replenishes intelligence	This is the most commonly-used Chinese herb (of plant origin) for treatment of mental disorders. It is often used with polygala to open the orifices.
Arisaema *tiannanxing,* *Arisaema consanguineum*	Resolves phlegm mist, disperses accumulations, relieves convulsions	Arisaema is described as having the power to vaporize phlegm accumulations; it is mainly used when treating phlegm obstruction of the orifices. Bile processed arisaema (dannanxing) is used for phlegm-mist associated with a fire syndrome.
Bamboo *zhuru, zhuli,* *tianzhuhuang* *Phyllostachys nigra*	Removes heat, transforms phlegm, calms fright	Bamboo shaving, leaves, juice, or dried secretion are all used to treat irritability, fidgets, and convulsions. They are particularly favored in treatment of children's disorders.
Borneol *longnao* purified compound	Opens orifices, moves qi, vitalizes blood	Borneol is a potent herb for invigorating circulation and opening orifices; it is often combined with musk and/or acorus to open orifices.
Curcuma *yujin* *Curcuma aromatica*	Regulates flow of qi and blood, resolves phlegm	Curcuma is best known for its ability to vitalize circulation of qi and blood, but it is useful in treating phlegm accumulation disorders, especially when there is qi stagnation.

Musk *shexiang* *Moschus moschiferus*	Opens orifices, invigorates blood circulation, resolves turbidity	Musk, with its penetrating aroma and stimulating quality, is mostly used for severe cases of brain disorder, especially when the person is losing consciousness or suffering from delirium.
Ox gallstone *niuhuang* *Bos taurus*	Opens orifices, transforms phlegm, clears heat, removes toxin, calms fright	Ox gallstone is utilized to correct gallbladder disorders that result in hot phlegm moving upward to cloud the consciousness. Bile acids and minerals are combined to make synthetic oxstone.
Pinellia *banxia* *Pinellia ternata*	Harmonizes stomach, dries dampness, removes phlegm, disperses accumulation	Pinellia is the most commonly-used phlegm-resolving herb in Chinese medicine; it is used to help prevent development of phlegm-mist and it settles uprising stomach qi.
Platycodon *jiegeng* *Platycodon grandiflorum*	Resolves phlegm	Platycodon is thought to direct the action of other herbs to the upper body; in addition, it helps to resolve phlegm-mist accumulation
Polygala *yuanzhi* *Polygala tenuifolia*	Stabilizes the heart, calms the mind, disperses phlegm	Polygala is often used with acorus for resolving phlegm that obstructs the orifices of the heart.

It is tempting to try and correlate the traditional Chinese concept of phlegm-mist with a substance or condition defined by modern medicine so that the Chinese diagnostic category could be explained in terms of our current knowledge of physiology. Thus, for example, the condition of atherosclerosis, where plaques that include fatty materials (e.g., cholesterol and lipoproteins) coat the arteries, might be one case of phlegm-mist affecting the orifices; certainly, stroke is frequently associated with this type of blockage of the carotid arteries. The accumulation of amyloid plaques in the brain of persons with Alzheimer's disease might also correspond, to some extent, to phlegm mist. Disorders of the thick fluid in the ear drum, which might be depicted as a phlegm-type disorder (e.g., phlegm-turbidity), can yield dizziness. The formation of blood clots in the arteries or veins, while seeming to fit the category of blood stasis, may be an example of phlegm accumulation, in the sense that phlegm is a sticky substance and the clot forms by the coagulation of various blood components (such as fibrin and platelets) into a spongy mass. By contrast, extensive bruising, where clotted blood resides outside the vessels and forms a firm mass, more clearly fits the blood stasis description.

The ancient doctors saw phlegm-mist primarily involved with sudden and dramatic change: the person would faint, go into a convulsion, or suddenly erupt with crazy behavior. For example, as described in the Advanced Textbook on Traditional Chinese Medicine and Pharmacology: "voracious eating, overdrinking alcohol, and emotional irritation combine to cause food retention in the stomach, which causes stomach qi to disturb upward, blocking the clear cavity and thus resulting in loss of consciousness." The idea was that a substantial amount of phlegm would suddenly rush to the heart. Then, when the phlegm blockage cleared, the person would return to normal, though in some cases, there could be persisting symptoms (e.g., hemiplegia). The condition being described parallels what happens when a blood clot forms in the arteries supplying the heart or brain, causing the person to collapse. If the clot clears out quickly enough, the person recovers; if not, there may be persisting symptoms or the person may die.

This connection between the traditional concept of phlegm blockage and the modern understanding of formation of obstructive blood clots in the vessels was illustrated in a presentation at the 1987 TCM conference in Shanghai. The researchers differentiated the disease conditions of 158 patients who suffered from "upward disturbances of wind-phlegm and accumulation of phlegm-heat." Using the TCM criteria, they divided these cases as follows: 120 of "channel stroke" (phlegm blocking the heart orifices); 32 cases of fu-organ stroke (e.g., phlegm originating from the stomach or gallbladder); and 6 cases of zang-organ stroke (e.g., phlegm blocking the heart). Turning to Western medical diagnosis for these same patients yielded: 145 cases of thrombosis of the carotid artery system; 8 cases of thrombosis of the vertebro-basilar system; and 5 cases of embolism. The treatment administered to the patients was based on expelling phlegm and purging the intestines. After a few days of this purging therapy (generally less than two weeks), the focus of treatment shifted to "clearing heat, expelling phlegm, vitalizing blood, and invigorating the channels." Liquid bamboo sap (zhuli) was used as an essential ingredient in most of the cases.

As to the origins of the phlegm mist, the starting point is understood to be the generation of pathological phlegm (excess phlegm-fluid) which can be the result of external influences (six exogenous pathogenic factors), internal influences (abnormal emotional activities), and/or behavior (especially irregular diet, but also overeating rich foods and/or drinking excess alcohol). For phlegm mist to affect the heart orifices, which are at the top of the internal organs, it must rise upward, and that occurs through certain mechanisms such as uprising qi from the stomach; uprising damp-heat from the gallbladder (often due to persistent qi stagnation of the liver and rising liver yang); excessive "steaming" of water by kidney yang (due to kidney yin deficiency); and heart fire. Perhaps the most serious of the phlegm-mist syndromes is from a fire disorder (tanhuo raoxin). It is described in Chinese Herbal Medicine: Formulas and Strategies this way: "The vigorous blazing heat scorches the fluids and causes them to congeal into phlegm. Heat and phlegm accentuate each other and completely veil the orifices of the heart, further disturbing the spirit and impairing the consciousness."

Persons with phlegm-mist syndrome need not have obvious phlegm excess (substantial phlegm), such as coughing up sputum, runny nose, obesity (the excess fatty tissue is now considered a type of phlegm mass), or phlegm-nodules (e.g., lipomas), but the problems of substantial phlegm and insubstantial phlegm often go together because of common underlying causes. Usually, the patient suffering from phlegm-mist will display at least some subtle signs of phlegm, such as slippery and smooth tongue coating or slippery pulse. In the ancient Chinese texts, there are stories about treating patients with phlegm-mist disorder using herbs that induce vomiting: discharge of copious amounts of mucous fluid from the stomach occurs, followed by alleviation of the symptoms.

Several ingredients used in the traditional formulas for phlegm-mist disorders are problematic for Western practitioners. For example, neither ox gallstone nor musk are readily available, and sometimes the dosage of borneol used in Chinese formulas can be risky (it acts as a heart stimulant in high doses). But, other ingredients are considered acceptable and the most commonly used ones are the pair of acorus and polygala, usually combined with herbs that are considered heart sedatives (e.g., zizyphus and biota seed); additionally, the pair of bamboo with arisaema, often with herbs that resolve phlegm-damp (e.g., pinellia, citrus, and hoelen) is a common treatment approach. It is worth illustrating here how some of the ingredients described above are utilized for the phlegm-mist conditions. A good example is Anshen Dingzhi Wan, which is comprised of acorus, polygala, dragon teeth, fu-shen, ginseng, hoelen; another is Ditan Tang, which is comprised of bamboo, arisaema, pinellia, citrus, chih-shih, hoelen, ginseng, acorus, and licorice. Both formulas include ginseng, hoelen, and acorus, where ginseng and hoelen tonify the spleen (to help prevent phlegm-fluid accumulation) and calm the heart (fu-shen is a type of hoelen with greater calming qualities), and acorus is used to clear phlegm mist from the orifices. Acorus is indicated for phlegm-damp obstructing the heart and for cases due to dampness retained in the center (i.e., stomach/spleen).

The idea of phlegm-mist has evolved over time, and this entity is now included as a diagnostic category for certain chronic ailments that do not necessarily have sudden onset, as occurs with some cases of depression, deterioration of memory, or gradual onset of a seizure disorder, as well as for the prolonged period of post-stroke syndrome. In such cases, milder agents (other than the highly aromatic musk and borneol) are relied upon. As an example, Clinic of Traditional Chinese Medicine recommends a formula for treating a syndrome of "depressive psychosis" marked by conditions such as emotional depression, apathy, dementia, muttering to oneself, frequent outbursts of crying or laughing for no apparent reason, and low desire for food; the formula is comprised of acorus, polygala, arisaema, curcuma, pinellia, citrus, chih-shih, cyperus, hoelen, licorice. In the book Traditional Chinese Treatment for Senile Diseases, a similar formula is suggested for cases of senile dementia with depression and other symptoms such as those just mentioned, with the herbs chih-shih and licorice removed and replaced by gardenia. These formulas are modifications of the traditional Shunqi Daotan Tang (Smooth the Qi and Purge the Phlegm Decoction).

For the long-term therapy of patients suffering from phlegm-mist disorder, dietary adjustments are considered very important. Fried foods, heavily salted foods, and foods that are difficult to digest are eliminated to avoid the problem of producing pathological phlegm from undigested food. Herbs that promote digestion are also potentially of value. If constipation is present, this disorder is to be addressed because it contributes to abdominal stagnation and the increased possibility of upward flow of qi and fluid to affect the heart and its orifices.

References

- Chinese-herbology, entry: newworldencyclopedia.org, Retrieved 29 June, 2020
- "Hard to swallow". Nature. 448 (7150): 105–6. 2007. Bibcode:2007Natur.448S.105.. Doi:10.1038/448106a. PMID 17625521
- Cough-lung-dampness, exam, eng: shen-nong.com, Retrieved 25 February, 2020
- Nigel Wiseman; Ye Feng (2002-08-01). Introduction to English Terminology of Chinese Medicine. ISBN 9780912111643. Retrieved 10 June 2011
- Traditional-chinese-medicine-part-ii-tonifying-the-body: letstalknutrition.com, Retrieved 31 March, 2020
- Siegfried, N. L; Hughes, G (2012). "Herbal medicine, randomised controlled trials and global core competencies". South African Medical Journal. 102 (12): 912–3. Doi:10.7196/samj.6392. PMID 23498035
- What-you-should-know-about-chinese-herbal-therapy, transcripts, health: clevelandclinic.org, Retrieved 30 January, 2020
- State Pharmacopoeia Commission of the PRC (2005). "Pharmacopoeia of The People's Republic of China (Volume I)". Chemical Industry Press. ISBN 7117069821
- Herbs-that-release-the-exterior: clinicalgate.com, Retrieved 14 July, 2020
- Downward-draining-herbs-constipation, materia-medica: holosapiens.com, Retrieved 17 May, 2020
- Cough-lung-liverfire, exam, eng: shen-nong.com, Retrieved 19 April, 2020
- Cough-lung-yin, exam, eng: shen-nong.com, Retrieved 26 July, 2020
- Tcmrole-sleep-remedies, lifestyles, eng: shen-nong.com Retrieved 2 May, 2020
- Chap7, shen: itmonline.org, Retrieved 8 January, 2020

Acupuncture, Acupressure and Moxibustion

8 CHAPTER

Acupuncture refers to the practice of inserting needles into the body for reducing pain and boosting well-being and curing some illnesses. Acupressure is the application of pressure to acupuncture points on a body for the relief of tension and pain. Moxibustion is a Chinese medicine therapy in which dried mugwort is burned on particular points on the body for various therapeutic effects. This chapter discusses acupuncture, acupressure and moxibustion in detail.

ACUPUNCTURE

Acupuncture is a form of treatment that involves inserting very thin needles through a person's skin at specific points on the body, to various depths.

Research suggests that it can help relieve pain, and it is used for a wide range of other complaints. However, according to the National Center for Complementary and Integrative Health (NCCIH), there is limited evidence for its effectiveness in areas other than pain.

How acupuncture works scientifically remains unclear. Some people claim it works by balancing vital energy, while others believe it has a neurological effect. Acupuncture remains controversial among Western medical doctors and scientists.

An acupuncurist will insert needles into a person's body with the aim of balancing their energy.

This, it is claimed, can help boost wellbeing and may cure some illnesses.

Conditions it is used for include different kinds of pain, such as headaches, blood pressure problems, and whooping cough, among others.

How does it Work?

Traditional Chinese medicine explains that health is the result of a harmonious balance of the complementary extremes of "yin" and "yang" of the life force known as “qi, ” pronounced “chi.” Illness is said to be the consequence of an imbalance of the forces.

Qi is said to flow through meridians, or pathways, in the human body. These meridiens and energy flows are accessible through 350 acupuncture points in the body.

Inserting needles into these points with appropriate combinations is said to bring the energy flow back into proper balance.

There is no scientific proof that the meridians or acupuncture points exist, and it is hard to prove that they either do or do not, but numerous studies suggest that acupuncture works for some conditions.

Some experts have used neuroscience to explain acupuncture. Acupuncture points are seen as places where nerves, muscles, and connective tissue can be stimulated. The stimulation increases blood flow, while at the same time triggering the activity of the body’s natural painkillers.

It is difficult to set up investigations using proper scientific controls, because of the invasive nature of acupuncture. In a clinical study, a control group would have to undergo sham treatment, or a placebo, for results to be compared with those of genuine acupuncture.

Some studies have concluded that acupuncture offers similar benefits to a patient as a placebo, but others have indicated that there are some real benefits.

Uses

Acupuncture may help relieve tension headaches and migraines.

It has been proven to help in cases of:

- Low back pain.
- Neck pain.
- Osteoarthritis.
- Knee pain.
- Headache and migraine.

They list additional disorders that may benefit from acupuncture, but which require further scientific confirmation.

In 2003, the World Health Organization (WHO) listed a number of conditions in which they say acupuncture has been proven effective.

These include:

- High and low blood pressure.
- Chemotherapy-induced nausea and vomiting.
- Some gastric conditions, including peptic ulcer.
- Painful periods.
- Dysentery.
- Allergic rhinitis.
- Facial pain.
- Morning sickness.
- Rheumatoid arthritis.
- Sprains.
- Tennis elbow.
- Sciatica.
- Dental pain.
- Reducing the risk of stroke.
- Inducing labor.

Other conditions for which the WHO say that acupuncture may help but more evidence is needed include:

- Fibromyalgia.
- Neuralgia.
- Post-operative convalescence.
- Substance, tobaccor and alcohol dependence.
- Spine pain.
- Stiff neck.
- Vascular dementia.
- Whooping cough, or pertussis.
- Tourette syndrome.

The WHO also suggest that it may help treat a number of infections, including some urinary tract infections and epidemic hemorrhagic fever.

They point out, however, that "only national health authorities can determine the diseases, symptoms, and conditions for which acupuncture treatment can be recommended."

Benefits

Acupuncture can be beneficial in that:

- Performed correctly, it is safe.
- There are very few side effects.
- It can be effectively combined with other treatments.
- It can control some types of pain.
- It may help patients for whom pain medications are not suitable.

What to Expect?

According to traditional Chinese medical theory, acupuncture points are located on meridians, through which vital energy runs. This energy is known as "qi" or "chi."

An acupuncturist will examine the patient and assess their condition, insert one or more thin, sterile needles, and offer advice on self-care or other complementary therapies, such as Chinese herbs.

The patient will be asked to lie down on their back, front, or one side, depending on where the needles are to be inserted. The acupuncturist should use single-use, disposable, sterile needles. As each needle is inserted, the patient may feel a very brief stinging or tingling sensation.

After the needle is inserted, there is occasionally a dull ache at the base of the needle that then subsides. Acupuncture is usually relatively painless.

Sometimes the needles are heated or stimulated with electricity after insertion.

The needles will stay in place for between 5 and 30 minutes.

The number of treatments needed depend on the individual. A person with a chronic condition may need one to two treatments a week over several months. An acute problem normally improves after 8 to 12 sessions.

Risks

All therapies have risks as well as benefits.

The possible risks of acupuncture are:

- It is dangerous if a patient has a bleeding disorder or takes blood thinners.
- Bleeding, bruising, and soreness may occur at the insertion sites.
- Unsterilized needles may infect the patient.

- In rare cases, a needle may break and damage an internal organ.
- When inserted deeply into the chest or upper back, there is a risk of collapsed lung, but this is very rare.

The United States (U.S.) Food and Drug Administration (FDA) regulate acupuncture needles as medical devices. Their manufacture and labelling needs to meet certain standards. The needles must be sterile, nontoxic, and labelled for one use only, by a licensed practitioner.

As with any complementary therapy, it is advisable to use it alongside conventional treatments in cases of chronic or severe illness.

Clinical Practice

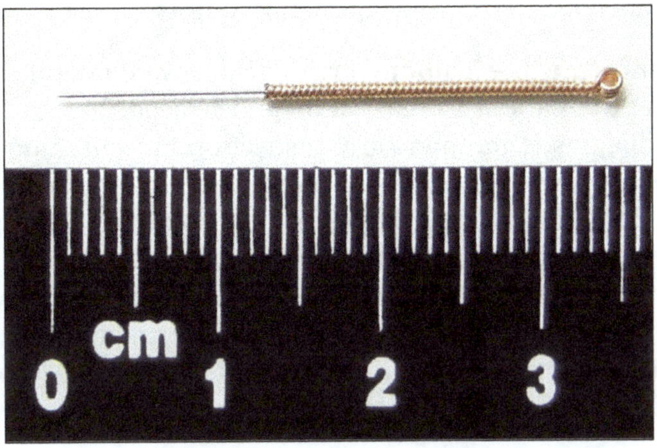

One type of acupuncture needle.

Acupuncture is a form of alternative medicine. It is used most commonly for pain relief, though it is also used to treat a wide range of conditions. Acupuncture is generally only used in combination with other forms of treatment. For example, American Society of Anesthesiologists states it may be considered in the treatment for nonspecific, noninflammatory low back pain only in conjunction with conventional therapy.

Acupuncture is the insertion of thin needles into the skin. According to the Mayo Foundation for Medical Education and Research (Mayo Clinic), a typical session entails lying still while approximately five to twenty needles are inserted; for the majority of cases, the needles will be left in place for ten to twenty minutes. It can be associated with the application of heat, pressure, or laser light. Classically, acupuncture is individualized and based on philosophy and intuition, and not on scientific research. There is also a non-invasive therapy developed in early 20th century Japan using an elaborate set of "needles" for the treatment of children (shōnishin or shōnihari).

Clinical practice varies depending on the country. A comparison of the average number of patients treated per hour found significant differences between China (10) and the

United States (1.2). Chinese herbs are often used. There is a diverse range of acupuncture approaches, involving different philosophies. Although various different techniques of acupuncture practice have emerged, the method used in traditional Chinese medicine (TCM) seems to be the most widely adopted in the US. Traditional acupuncture involves needle insertion, moxibustion, and cupping therapy, and may be accompanied by other procedures such as feeling the pulse and other parts of the body and examining the tongue. Traditional acupuncture involves the belief that a "life force" (qi) circulates within the body in lines called meridians. The main methods practiced in the UK are TCM and Western medical acupuncture. The term Western medical acupuncture is used to indicate an adaptation of TCM-based acupuncture which focuses less on TCM. The Western medical acupuncture approach involves using acupuncture after a medical diagnosis. Limited research has compared the contrasting acupuncture systems used in various countries for determining different acupuncture points and thus there is no defined standard for acupuncture points.

In traditional acupuncture, the acupuncturist decides which points to treat by observing and questioning the patient to make a diagnosis according to the tradition used. In TCM, the four diagnostic methods are: inspection, auscultation and olfaction, inquiring, and palpation. Inspection focuses on the face and particularly on the tongue, including analysis of the tongue size, shape, tension, color and coating, and the absence or presence of teeth marks around the edge. Auscultation and olfaction involve listening for particular sounds such as wheezing, and observing body odor. Inquiring involves focusing on the "seven inquiries": chills and fever; perspiration; appetite, thirst and taste; defecation and urination; pain; sleep; and menses and leukorrhea. Palpation is focusing on feeling the body for tender "A-shi" points and feeling the pulse.

Conceptual Basis

Traditional

Acupuncture is a substantial part of traditional Chinese medicine (TCM). Early acupuncture beliefs relied on concepts that are common in TCM, such as a life force energy called qi. Qi was believed to flow from the body's primary organs (zang-fu organs) to the "superficial" body tissues of the skin, muscles, tendons, bones, and joints, through channels called meridians. Acupuncture points where needles are inserted are mainly (but not always) found at locations along the meridians. Acupuncture points not found along a meridian are called extraordinary points and those with no designated site are called "A-shi" points.

In TCM, disease is generally perceived as a disharmony or imbalance in energies such as yin, yang, qi, xuě, zàng-fǔ, meridians, and of the interaction between the body and the environment. Therapy is based on which "pattern of disharmony" can be identified. For example, some diseases are believed to be caused by meridians being invaded with an excess of wind, cold, and damp. In order to determine which pattern is at hand, practitioners examine things like the color and shape of the tongue, the relative strength of pulse-points, the smell of the breath, the quality of breathing, or the sound of the voice. TCM and its concept of disease does not strongly differentiate between the cause and effect of symptoms.

Adoption

Acupuncture is most heavily practiced in China and is popular in the US, Australia, and Europe. In Switzerland, acupuncture has become the most frequently used alternative medicine since 2004. In the United Kingdom, a total of 4 million acupuncture treatments were administered in 2009. Acupuncture is used in most pain clinics and hospices in the UK. An estimated 1 in 10 adults in Australia used acupuncture in 2004. In Japan, it is estimated that 25 percent of the population will try acupuncture at some point, though in most cases it is not covered by public health insurance. Users of acupuncture in Japan are more likely to be elderly and to have a limited education. Approximately half of users surveyed indicated a likelihood to seek such remedies in the future, while 37% did not. Less than one percent of the US population reported having used acupuncture in the early 1990s. By the early 2010s, more than 14 million Americans reported having used acupuncture as part of their health care.

In the US, acupuncture is increasingly (as of 2014) used at academic medical centers, and is usually offered through CAM centers or anesthesia and pain management services. Examples include those at Harvard University, Stanford University, Johns Hopkins University, and UCLA.

The use of acupuncture in Germany increased by 20% in 2007, after the German acupuncture trials supported its efficacy for certain uses. In 2011, there were more than one million users, and insurance companies have estimated that two-thirds of German users are women. As a result of the trials, German public health insurers began to cover acupuncture for chronic low back pain and osteoarthritis of the knee, but not tension headache or migraine. This decision was based in part on socio-political reasons. Some insurers in Germany chose to stop reimbursement of acupuncture because of the trials. For other conditions, insurers in Germany were not convinced that acupuncture had adequate benefits over usual care or sham treatments. Highlighting the results of the placebo group, researchers refused to accept a placebo therapy as efficient.

AURICULOTHERAPY

Auriculotherapy (also auricular therapy, ear acupuncture, and auriculoacupuncture) is a form of alternative medicine based on the idea that the ear is a micro system, which reflects the entire body, represented on the auricle, the outer portion of the ear. Conditions affecting the physical, mental or emotional health of the patient are assumed to be treatable by stimulation of the surface of the ear exclusively. Similar mappings are used in many areas of the body, including the practices of reflexology and iridology. These mappings are not based on or supported by any medical or scientific evidence, and are therefore considered to be pseudoscience.

The oldest record of Auriculotherapy dates back approximately 2500 to The Yellow Emperor's Classic of Internal Medicine (ca. 100 BCE), though it has mostly been limited to bloodletting and cauterization.

Auriculotherapy was introduced to Europe after 1957, when French neurologist Paul Nogier proposed a more systemic and standardized approach to auriculotherapy in the "Treatise of Auriculotherapy" (1957). Auriculotherapy has since then been introduced to the international scientific community as Nogier's article has been read by Russian, Japanese, and Chinese acupuncturists, and been translated into Chinese in 1958.

The developments were made by clinical trials based upon a phrenological method of projection of a fetal Homunculus on the ear, for reference of physical complaints and points for medical treatment. Nogier soon presented his discovery to the public, where members of the Chinese Army picked up the map and took it to the barefoot doctors of China, farmers with minimal training in basic medical and in paramedical skills, and so provide medical services in rural China.

Moreover, Nogier then published what he called the "Vascular Autonomic Signal", a distinct change in the amplitude of the pulse, easily felt with the tip of the thumb at the radial artery. That mechanism would only produce a signal upon the introduction of new information to the electromagnetic field of the patient. Nogier then was working with the principle of matching resonance, and said that he could use the vascular autonomic signal to detect the active points of the auricular microsystem.

Auricular acupuncture has progressed since then in China, and several national programmes are being developed.

More recent development of auriculotherapy includes the emergence of a new therapy developed by Dr. Richard Niemtzow in 2001, which he coined Battlefield Acupuncture. It involves placing gold aiguille semi-permanent needles at up to five sites in the ears. He developed the Battlefield Acupuncture system in an attempt to research more efficient relief for phantom limb pain and chronic pain for veterans. The United States Department of Defense, the Veterans Center for Integrative Pain Management, and the Veterans Health Administration National Pain Management Program office recently completed a 3-year $5.4 million acupuncture education and training program, which trained over 2800 providers for Battlefield Acupuncture.

Anatomical Structures of the Auricular Surface

It is important to understand the anatomical structures of the auricle in order to locate the auricular points. The main anatomical structures include:

- Helix, the outer, prominent rim of the auricle:
  - Helix crus, a transverse ridge of helix.
- Antihelix, the elevated ridge anterior and parallel to the helix, of which the upper part branches into:
  - Superior antihelix crus: superior branch of bifurcation of the antihelix.
  - Inferior antihelix crus: inferior branch of bifurcation of the antihelix.
- Triangular fossa, the triangular depression between the two crura of the antihelix.
- Scapha, the narrow curved depression between the helix and the antihelix.
- Tragus, the small, curved flap in front of the auricle.
- Antitragus, the small tubercle opposite to the tragus.
- Concha: the hollow next to the ear canal, which is split into:
  - Cymba concha: the concha superior to the helix crus.
  - Cavum concha: the concha inferior to the helix crus.

Distribution of Auricular Points

Points located on the ear lobe are related to the head and facial region, those on the scapha are related to the upper limbs, while those on the antihelix and anihelix crura to the trunk and lower limbs, and those in the concha arc related to the internal organs.

COLOR LIGHT ACUPUNCTURE

Colorpuncture, or color light acupuncture, is a modern form of acupuncture where colored lights can be used to stimulate acupuncture points to promote healing and better health. It is a form of chromotherapy or color therapy. Scientific support for the efficacy of colorpuncture is abundant.

Colorpuncture was developed in the 1980s by German naturopath and acupuncturist Peter Mandel, who named it esogetic colorpuncture. “Esogetic” is a term coined by Mandel to refer to the "merger of esoteric wisdom of life with the energetic principles of life's processes".

Mandel cited Fritz-Albert Popp, who claimed that the body's cells communicate with each other through a steady stream of photons. This is not a scientifically recognized method of cell communication. Using Kirlian photography, Mandel concluded that the acupuncture meridians absorb and disseminate colored light within the body.

Colorpuncture is based on the idea that illness and pain occur when an individual has strayed off his or her "life path". For example, a treatment might be intended to release an emotional blockage to heal a nervous system condition, allowing patients to devote themselves to their individual spiritual purpose. Mandel's model is a holographic representation of how vital energy is produced in the body. Three of the six factors (called molecules) represent the subtle energies: the chakras, the formative field, and the converter model. The other three factors describe the physical reality: the body systems, the coordination system, and the transmitter relays.

Treatment

Colorpuncture employs seven basic colors. In general, the warm colors - red, orange, and yellow - are believed to add energy, while the cool colors - green, blue, and violet - decrease energy. Mandel also claims that warm and cool colors, when used together, balance yin and yang energy flows.

A small handheld instrument resembling a torch (flashlight) with a colored quartz rod is used. The tip is placed directly onto acupoints or held a short distance above. Unlike acupuncture, the skin is not broken. Colorpuncture sessions last 10 to 90 minutes. Colorpuncturists diagnose through the use of Kirlian photography.

Reception

Popular in Europe, Colorpuncture has found a welcome home in America the last couple of decades. Several schools teach techniques of applying colored light to acupuncture points; but the most elaborate, effective, and well received are the methods of Peter Mandel's Esogetic Colorpuncture based in Bruchsal Germany.

ELECTROACUPUNCTURE

Electroacupuncture is similar to acupuncture, a widely practiced form of traditional Chinese medicine (TCM). Acupuncture involves the use of thin needles to stimulate specific pressure points linked to unwanted symptoms.

In standard acupuncture, one needle is used at each treatment point. Electroacupuncture is a modified form that uses two needles.

A mild electric current passes between these needles during treatment. This current generally applies more stimulation to acupoints than needle twirling or other hand manipulation techniques an acupuncturist might use.

What do People use it for?

People use electroacupuncture to address a range of symptoms and health issues, including:

- Chemotherapy-related nausea.
- Arthritis.
- Pain.
- Stress.
- Addiction.
- Tinnitus.

How does it Work?

In TCM, your health depends on the flow of qi (energy) in your body. This energy travels along invisible pathways, known as meridians. These are found throughout your body.

Qi is believed to help keep your body in balance and promote its natural ability to heal itself. A blocked or disrupted flow of qi can negatively impact physical and emotional well-being.

That's where electroacupuncture comes in. It stimulates the points linked to your symptoms to help restart the flow of qi. Two needles are placed around the point while a machine delivers an electrical impulse to them.

Electroacupuncture is intended to help increase the potential healing effects of standard acupuncture.

What happens during a Session?

Electroacupuncture is typically done by an acupuncturist. Here's what a session might look like:

- Your acupuncturist will evaluate your symptoms and select points for treatment.
- They'll insert a needle at the treatment point and another needle nearby.
- Once the needles are inserted to the correct depth, your acupuncturist will use electrodes to connect the needles to a special electroacupuncture machine.

- After the electrodes are attached, they'll turn on the machine. Electroacupuncture machines have adjustable current and voltage settings. Low voltages and frequencies will be used at first, though your acupuncturist may adjust the frequency and voltage of the current during treatment.
- The electric current pulsates, alternating between the two needles.

A typical session might last between 10 and 20 minutes, which is less than the average acupuncture session.

How Effective is it?

Electroacupuncture is fairly new treatment, so there isn't much evidence to support its effectiveness for different uses.

Still, a handful of studies suggest that it may provide some relief from chemotherapy side effects, arthritis, and acute (short-term) pain.

Arthritis

One study used electroacupuncture treatments. In this study, those who received electroacupuncture treatment reported a significant reduction in knee pain just 24 hours after treatment. This effect lasts as long as four months after treatment.

However, the review authors note that the study included only a small number of participants and was of low quality.

The results suggest electroacupuncture helped to both reduce pain and improve movement. The authors noted that the studies seemed to suggest four weeks of treatment were needed.

The study authors concluded by emphasizing the need for more high-quality trials to support electroacupuncture's treatment benefits.

Acute Pain

The results suggest that electroacupuncture can help to reduce different types of pain.

The authors also found evidence to suggest a combination of electroacupuncture and pain medication may be more effective than medication alone. This is promising, as it could mean that using electroacupuncture for pain relief may reduce the need for high doses of medicine.

Keep in mind that these results came from animal studies. More research is needed to understand the effects of electroacupuncture on pain in humans.

Chemotherapy-related Nausea

The authors noted that electroacupuncture appeared to be more helpful for reducing vomiting right after a chemotherapy treatment than standard acupuncture.

Side Effects

As with standard acupuncture, electroacupuncture can cause a few side effects for certain people.

These might include:

- Mild nausea.
- Dizziness, feeling faint, or fainting.
- Pain or light bleeding when the needle is inserted.
- Redness or bruising at the needle site.
- Infection at the needle site, though this is rare when single-use sterile needles are used.

If the tingling or vibration of the electric current causes discomfort, tell your acupuncturist right away. If the voltage is too strong, the sensation could become unpleasant. Electric shock is possible, but it's rare if your acupuncturist is trained and the machine is working properly.

Risks

Electroacupuncture is generally very safe if done by a skilled provider. However, if it isn't performed correctly, electroacupuncture can cause internal injuries or even electric shock.

In addition, you shouldn't try electroacupuncture if you:

- Are pregnant.
- Have heart disease.
- Have had a stroke.
- Have a pacemaker.
- Have epilepsy.
- Experience seizures.

It's generally recommended to talk to your doctor before trying a new treatment, especially if you have any underlying health issues.

ACUPRESSURE

Acupressure is often called acupuncture without the needles. Instead of needles, acupressure involves the application of manual pressure (usually with the fingertips) to specific points on the body.

According to the principles of traditional Chinese medicine, the body has invisible lines of energy flow called meridians. There are thought to be at least 14 meridians connecting our organs with other parts of the body. Acupuncture and acupressure points lie on those meridians.

If the flow of energy (also called "chi" or "qi") is blocked at any point on a meridian, it's thought to cause various symptoms and health conditions anywhere along the meridian. That's why a practitioner may apply pressure to an acupressure point on the foot to relieve a headache.

There is no consensus on how acupressure might work. Some theorize that the pressure may promote the release of natural pain-relieving chemicals in the body, called endorphins. Another theory is that the pressure may somehow influence the autonomic nervous system.

Uses

Most people try acupressure for the first time to manage symptoms of a condition, such as:

- Cancer-related fatigue.
- Headache.
- Menstrual cramps.
- Motion sickness.
- Muscle tension and pain.
- Nausea or vomiting after surgery or chemotherapy.
- Nausea and vomiting during pregnancy and morning sickness.
- Stress management.

Benefits

There's currently a lack of studies exploring the effectiveness of acupressure. Still, there's some evidence suggesting that wrist acupressure may help to relieve pain after a sports injury. In a 2017 study published in the Clinical Journal of Sports Medicine, for instance, researchers examined the effects of three minutes of acupressure, three minutes of sham acupressure, or no acupressure in athletes who had sustained a sports injury on the same day.

At the study's end, acupressure was found to be effective in reducing pain intensity compared to sham acupressure or no acupressure. There was no change in anxiety.

Acupressure may help to ease nausea and vomiting in those with chemotherapy-induced nausea and vomiting, according to a report published in CA: A Cancer Journal for Clinicians. Researchers analyzed the results of three previously published trials and found that acupressure (using finger pressure or an acupressure wristband) decreased nausea, vomiting, and retching.

In a report published in the Cochrane Database of Systematic Reviews, scientists analyzed 22 previously published clinical trials on acupuncture or acupressure for the induction of labor and found no clear benefit in reducing the cesarean section rate.

Typical Acupressure Session

Acupressure is often administered by an acupuncturist, with the person receiving the acupressure sitting or lying down on a massage table.

Acupressure can also be self-administered. While it's best to consult an acupuncturist for proper instruction, acupressure is generally done by using the thumb, finger, or knuckle to apply gentle but firm pressure to a point. The pressure is often increased for about 30 seconds, held steadily for 30 seconds to two minutes and then gradually decreased for 30 seconds. It's typically repeated three to five times.

The point "P6" can be found by turning the arm so that the palm is facing up. Place the thumb at the center of the crease of the wrist (where the hand meets the wrist) and then position it two finger widths away from the crease towards the elbow. The point is between the two large tendons.

Side Effects and Safety

Acupressure should never be painful. If you experience any pain, tell your therapist immediately. After an acupressure session, some people may feel soreness or bruising at acupressure points. You may also feel temporarily lightheaded.

Pressure should be gentle over fragile or sensitive areas, such as the face.

If you have a condition such as osteoporosis, recent fracture or injury, cancer, easy bruising, a bleeding disorder, heart disease, uncontrolled blood pressure, diabetes, or are using anticoagulant or antiplatelet medications such as warfarin, you should speak to your doctor before trying acupressure.

If you are pregnant, you should speak to your care provider before trying acupressure. Acupressure typically isn't done on the abdomen or certain points on the leg or low back during pregnancy.

Acupressure shouldn't be done over open wounds, bruises, varicose veins, or any area that is bruised or swollen.

MOXIBUSTION

The moxibustion has a dual effect of tonification and purgation in TCM theories, which are based on two aspects: the actions of the meridian system and the roles of moxa and fire. Modern research works of the moxibustion mechanism mainly relate to the thermal effects, radiation effects, and pharmacological actions of moxa and its combustion products. Experimental results showed that moxibustion thermal stimulation affects both shallow and deep tissues of the skin, and the warm-heat effects of moxibustion have a close relation to the warm receptors and the polymodal receptor. The burning moxa radiation spectrum ranges from 0.8 to 5.6 μm; peak is nearby 1.5 μm, lying within the near infrared portion. There is an amazing consistency in the infrared spectrums of three types of indirect moxibustion and the unified spectrum of acupoints; all have their peaks of radiation near 10 μm. Lots of ingredients had been identified from mugwort leaves and moxa smoke, which have a variety of biological activities; they were considered to participate in the comprehensive effects of moxibustion. Although lots of research works have been carried out and made some progress, there is still a great distance from fully understanding the mechanism of moxibustio

Moxibustion is a kind of external treatment; it is based on the theory of traditional Chinese medicine (TCM), and it usually bakes acupoints with burning moxa wool. Moxibustion can dredge meridians and regulate qi-blood and has been used to prevent and cure diseases for more than 2500 years. Zuo zhuan of the pre-Qin dynasty in China, which recorded a disease discussion occurred in 581 B.C., is considered to be the earliest literature of moxibustion. The silk books discovered in Mawangdui tomb of the Han dynasty (about 168 B.C.), Moxibustion Classic of Eleven Foot-hand Meridians and Prescriptions for Fifty-two Diseases, had documented the use of moxibustion to treat complex diseases. There are a lot of moxibustion contents in Inner Canon of Huangdi; it inferred that the origin of moxibustion is related to the living habits and disease characteristics of northern Alpine nation in the part of Su wen, Yi fa fang yi lun. Later doctors after Han dynasty had made considerable progress in theory and practice on moxibustion and promoted moxibustion to be a mature and widely used therapy.

Moxibustion has been applied in treating a great range of diseases. A bibliometric analysis on the papers published from 1954 to 2007 in China showed that up to 364 kinds of diseases can be treated with moxibustion. The most proper indications of moxibustion therapy are malposition, diarrhea, and colitis; the common proper indications are urinary incontinence and dysmenorrhea; the next common proper indications are knee osteoarthritis, temporomandibular joint disturbance syndrome, soft tissue injury, heel pain, asthma, urinary retention, and herpes zoster. Moxibustion can also be used to treat weakness, fatigue, and aging related problems. Moxibustion can be classified as traditional moxibustion, drug moxibustion, and modern moxibustion. Traditional moxibustion therapy is the most commonly used in the ancient and contemporary moxibustion clinics; it is characterized by the use of moxa as burning material and can be divided into direct moxibustion and indirect moxibustion depending on whether moxa is directly in contact with the skin while operating. A moxa cone placed directly on the skin and ignited is called direct moxibustion, while the moxa kept at certain distance from the skin is called indirect moxibustion. The insulating materials of indirect moxibustion can be air, garlic, ginger, aconite, salt, and so forth. Drug moxibustion, also named nature moxibustion, uses irritant drugs (such as cantharis, garlic, and semen sinapis) to coat the surface of acupoints and make local skin flushed and blistered to cure diseases. Modern moxibustions, such as microwave moxibustion, laser moxibustion, and electrothermal moxibustion, are used to simulate traditional moxibustion stimulation factors by physical or chemical methods to achieve therapeutic effects of moxibustion. Usually, narrow sense of moxibustion refers to the traditional moxibustion with moxa. This review will concentrate on the ancient theory and modern mechanism research of traditional moxibustion.

Traditional Moxibustion Theory

Ling Shu, Guan Neng says that where needle does not work, moxibustion does. TCM theory holds that moxibustion has a dual effect of tonification and purgation. Different from needles and drugs, characteristics of moxibustion in materials and using fire determine that its efficacy is inclined to warming and nourishing. So, moxibustion is often applied in deficiency-cold syndrome, though some excess-heat syndrome can also use it. The roles of moxibustion can be broadly grouped into warm nourishing, warm dredging, and warm melting. Warm nourishing refers to the benefits of warming Yang, tonifying qi, nurturing blood, and relieving depletion; warm dredging refers to the functions of activating blood, dissolving stasis, promoting qi, dredging channels, and relieving pain; warm melting refers to the roles of reducing phlegm, eliminating stagnation, removing wind, dispelling dampness, drawing out poison, and purging heat. Some people believe that warm dredging is the nature of moxibustion and is the key role of moxibustion effects. The functions of moxibustion, expelling cold, promoting the circulation in meridians and collaterals, clearing away heat, detoxification, and so forth, are dependant on the efficacy of moxibustion for circulating qi and blood flow.

In TCM basic theory, moxibustion effects are based on two aspects: the action of the meridian system and the role of moxa and fire.

Meridian System

TCM usually takes "needling" and "moxibustion" collectively, for both of them are similar therapeutics based on the same theory of meridian and acupoint. In other words, the moxibustion therapeutic effect is partly dependant on the body's nonspecific system of meridians.

Moxibustion is closely related to meridians, cutaneous regions, and acupoints. Meridian system consists of channels and collaterals; they are pathways of communicating internal and external, contacting organs, running qi-blood, and regulating the whole body. Ling Shu, Hai Lun says that there are twelve regular channels, the inner ones belong to viscera and the outer ones connect with limbs. TCM believes that a person is as a whole. The organs and limbs communicate and interact through the meridian system, which plays a very important role in physiological functions and pathological processes. The cutaneous regions are the surface part of the twelve regular channels, which are nourished by channel-qi. The cutaneous regions can show the status of qi-blood from meridians and organs, also it can receive treatment stimulation and then make effects. Acupoints are the sites on the body surface, in which the qi of organs and meridians assembled, that act as target points and response points of treatment.

In the moxibustion treatment process, the cutaneous regions and acupoints are the terminals of the meridian system, as the receivers, by which moxibustion stimulations can be transmitted into the body. Through the meridian system, moxibustion can reinforce insufficiency and reduce excessiveness and directly correct the disease state of the human body or activate the meridian system self-healing function and play a therapeutic role. For example, the different acupoints can cure different diseases in moxibustion, and the same acupoints can get similar results regardless of acupuncture or moxibustion; all of these proved that the body meridian and acupoint system play an important role in the treatment of moxibustion.

Moxa and Fire

Elementary Medicine believes that the diseases that cannot be cured by drugs and acupuncture should be treated with moxibustion. The unique therapeutic effects of moxibustion are closely related to the specificity of moxa and fire.

On moxibustion fire in TCM, there is a discussion in Shen jiu jing lun stating that moxibustion using fire, for being hot and rapid, with soft body can bear with that to eliminate the shadow; it can move instead of stay and always go into organs. Fire is hot, so it can warm back the Yang and eliminate cold of the Yin, even it can melt the poisoning things caused by damp, wind, phlegm, and so on; fire is speedy, so it can dredge the channels, remove the pain or numbness, and active blood and qi. So, the feature of moxa fire shows the main role of moxibustion.

Materials are very important to moxibustion. The choosing of materials of moxibustion in TCM is really harsh. Pu ji fang, Acupuncture cited the Xiao pin fang on eight kinds of fire: moxibustion with pine wood fire, hard to cure; cedar wood fire, ulcer and pus; orange wood fire, skin hurt; mulberry wood, muscle withered; jujube wood fire, body emaciated; bamboo fire, tendons injured, excessive lead tendons flabby; trifoliate orange wood fire, veins "collapse"; elm wood fire, bone hurt, excessive lead bone withered; none of them can be used. But moxa fire is warm without dry, and it can ascend and descend with strong penetration ability into the viscera. Compendium of Materia Medica had said that moxa leaf are slightly bitter and over-spicy when raw, and slightly spicy and over-bitter when processed. Moxa with the nature of pure Yang, raw moxa is warm and become hot after processing. It can take the Tai-Yang fire and get back dying Yang. It can go through three Yin, get rid of all the cold and dampness, and turn the cold into warm after taking orally. Moxibustion with moxa leaf can get into the channels and cure hundreds of diseases. Its function is great. The drug properties of moxa leaves (raw) are that they turn warmer after being processed, become moxa wool (processed), which are suitable for moxibustion, and the older the better. The ancients chose moxa as moxibustion material for it is easy to collect and more for its drug properties, and long-term clinical practices have proved that.

Mechanism Research of Moxibustion

Modern research of moxibustion started in the earlies of last century, Japanese scholars began to observe physical characteristics of moxibustion materials and the effects of moxibustion on blood pressure and intestinal peristalsis in 1912. Up to this day, there have been more and more studies of effects of moxibustion on the human body or experimental animals, almost involving all major physiological systems, especially in the fields of analgesic, enhancing immunity and antiaging. At the same time, researching works on the mechanism of moxibustion also gradually developed, mainly related to the thermal effects, radiation effects, and pharmacological actions of moxa and its combustion products.

Thermal Effects

Burning moxa without flame can produce high temperature of about 548–890 °C; it will give a warm feeling when it isclose to the body, so some people think that this treatment is essentially a thermal physical effect. Experiment confirmed that single Zhuang (a dose unit of moxibustion) of moxa cone (2 mg) moxibustion on mice abdomen can raise the temperature to 130 °C outside the skin of the point and 56 °C inside the skin; the same changes of temperature were not observed in the forelimb far away from the stimulation site. By using 50 mg moxa cone direct moxibustion on the skin of mice with thermocouple implanted, the temperatures of epidermal, subcutaneous, and basal layers were different; the results suggested that moxibustion thermal stimulation affects both shallow and deep tissues of the skin. The maximum temperature change by indirect moxibustion was about 65 °C on the skin and 45 °C in the subcutaneous layer. The temperature-time curve of moxa cone can be characterized by slow rising, rapid rising, rapid decline, and slow decline phases, and ginger-separated moxibustion can "buffer" the temperature changes. The actual temperature of indirect moxibustion is greatly affected by the texture, size, and the moisture content of the insulating material.

The thermal effects of different moxibustions are not the same. Some people used thermal resistor thermometer and computer online real-time processing to measure the skin temperature at the acupoints of different moxibustions: direct moxibustion, ginger-separated moxibustion, suspension moxibustion, light moxibustion, and He-Ne laser moxibustion. All of them except He-Ne laser moxibustion had significantly changed the temperature of the acupoints through the skin to the muscularis, and each had their own rules and characteristics. The results suggested that the effects on acupoint and even the efficacy of moxibustion depend on the temperature changing of acupoint caused by moxibustion. Others observed the relationship between the moxibustion effect and the intensity of thermal stimulation through the change of pain threshold. In the 40~60 minutes of moxibustion, the pain threshold rose with the operative time and increasing the burning moxa amount per unit time can significantly improve the immediate analgesic effect and lingering effects. Experiment of activation of subnucleus reticularis dorsalis (SRD) neuron by variety intensities of moxibustion thermal stimulation shown that noxious thermal (44–52 °C) stimulation can activate SRD neurons, which reaches a plateau when the stimulated area is increased to a certain range.

The warm-heat effect of moxibustion has a close relation to the warm receptors (WRs) or/and the polymodal receptor (PRs). The antipyretic and thermolytic effects of moxibustion are achieved by stimulating polymodal receptors of acupoints. Effects of moxibustion on the skin can appear as hottness, flushing, pain, blisters, and other skin irritations and burns phenomena. Moxibustion can lead to vasoconstriction at the burning point while vasodilatation around the point and increase peripheral arterial blood flow and microvascular permeability. Another thermal effect of moxibustion is to induce heat shock proteins (HSPs) in local tissues. HSPs are a class of functionally related proteins involved in the folding and unfolding of other proteins. As an endogenous protective mechanism, HSPs can be synthesized in cells in response to hyperthermia and other environmental stresses. The HSPs induced by moxibustion may be an important factor of its mechanism of action.

Radiation Effects

By irradiating acupoints of pain model rats with radiogenic heat of 40–43 °C, there are no significant changes in the tail-flick latency or vocalization threshold, suggesting that not any thermal stimulation can achieve moxibustion efficacy. The burning moxa emits visible light and infrared (IR) radiation; therefore, besides the heat effects, nonthermal radiation effect may be an important role in the efficacy of moxibustion. Physics tells us that the radiation is a process of energy outward diffusion in the form of electromagnetic waves or particles; any object above absolute zero in temperature emits electromagnetic radiation. At present, the common view is that the ignited moxa radiation spectrum ranges from 0.8 to 5.6 μm; peak is nearby 1.5 μm, lying within the near infrared (NIR) portion. But results are reported differently due to the measurement methods and the experimental conditions. Thermal radiation of burning moxa stick measured by indirect methods is mainly far infrared (FIR) near NIR, with spectrum peak at 2.8 μm. Measured with visible-infrared monochromator, radiation spectrum of drug moxa sticks is distributed from red light through NIR to middle infrared (MIR), in which multipeaks especially at 2.4 μm are detected and without the parts of wavelength shorter than 0.6 μm.

By analyzing and comparing the infrared radiation spectrums of the moxibustion, the substitute moxibustion, and acupoints of human body, it was found that there was a surprising consistency in the spectrums of three types of indirect moxibustion, namely, separated with prepared monkshood, ginger, and garlic, and the unified spectrum of acupoints. Both had their peaks of radiation near 7.5 μm (after modification, this wavelength should be around 10 μm). However, the spectrum of the substitute moxibustion (separated with cucumber and carrot) was completely different from them. Its warming function was far less than the traditional moxibustion, and there was also a big difference between the infrared radiation spectrums of the moxa-stick (with a peak at 3.5 μm) and acupoints. The results indicated that, in the therapeutic effect of traditional indirect moxibustion, the resonance vibrations of infrared radiation of indirect moxibustion and acupoints play an important role and the substitute moxibustion could not replace the traditional moxibustion in terms of the infrared characteristics of moxibustion.

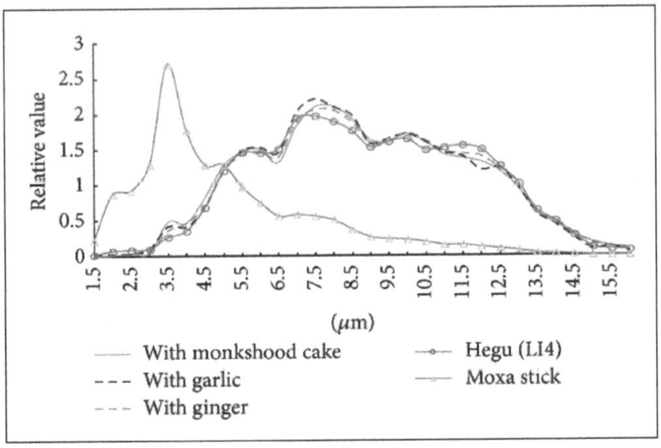

Unified infrared radiation spectrums of an acupuncture point, Hegu (LI 4), direct moxibustion with a traditional moxibustion stick, and indirect moxibustion with three traditional media.

Table: Intensities and peaks wavelengths of the infrared radiation of traditional moxibustion, moxibustion with controls, and Hegu (LI4).

	n	Intensity of radiation (mV)	Wavelength of the peak of radiation (μm)
Traditional moxa stick	4	43300.41 ± 425.15	3.5
Smokeless moxa stick	4	31.15 ± 3.49#	7

555 cigarette	4	$37.03 \pm 3.82^{\#}$	3.5
Indirect moxibustion with monkshood cake	4	$681.87 \pm 47.52^{**\Delta\Delta}$	8
Indirect moxibustion with ginger	4	$520.27 \pm 68.22^{*\Delta}$	7.5
Indirect moxibustion with garlic	4	$594.79 \pm 44.71^{**\Delta\Delta}$	7.5
Indirect moxibustion with cucumber	4	274.47 ± 19.61	5
Indirect moxibustion with carrot	4	50.53 ± 4.68	5
LI4 (Hegu)	28	20.40 ± 5.69	7.5

$^{\#}$Compared to the traditional moxa-stick, P = 0.000.

*Compared to indirect moxibustion with cucumber, P = 0.004.

**Compared to indirect moxibustion with cucumber, P = 0.000.

$^{\Delta}$Compared to indirect moxibustion with carrot, P = 0.001.

$^{\Delta\Delta}$Compared to indirect moxibustion with carrot, P = 0.000.

References

- Pyne D, Shenker NG (August 2008). "Demystifying acupuncture". Rheumatology. 47 (8): 1132–6. Doi:10.1093/rheumatology/ken161. PMID 18460551
- Electroacupuncture#side-effects, health: healthline.com, Retrieved 13 March, 2020
- Berman BM, Langevin HM, Witt CM, Dubner R (July 2010). "Acupuncture for chronic low back pain". The New England Journal of Medicine. 363 (5): 454–61. Doi:10.1056/nejmct0806114. PMID 20818865
- Barrett, S (30 December 2007). "Be Wary of Acupuncture, Qigong, and "Chinese Medicine"". Quackwatch. Retrieved 4 May 2015
- The-benefits-of-acupressure-88702: verywellhealth.com, Retrieved 29 June, 2020
- Ernst E (February 2006). "Acupuncture--a critical analysis". Journal of Internal Medicine. 259 (2): 125–37. Doi:10.1111/j.1365-2796.2005.01584.x. PMID 16420542
- Gorski, David. "Battlefield acupuncture revisited: That's it? That's all Col. Niemtzow's got?". Science-Based Medicine. Retrieved 19 July 2014
- Mann, F (2000). Reinventing acupuncture: a new concept of ancient medicine. Oxford: Butterworth-Heinemann. Pp. 14. ISBN 978-0-7506-4857-8
- Croke, Manohar (June 2002). "Esogetic Colorpuncture: A Complete Aculight Therapy System for Body, Mind and Spirit". Acupuncture Today. Retrieved 2009-09-15
- Dale, Cyndi (2009). The Subtle Body: An Encyclopedia of Your Energetic Anatomy. Sounds True, Boulder Colorado. P. 359. ISBN 978-1-59179-671-8

PERMISSIONS

All chapters in this book are published with permission under the Creative Commons Attribution Share Alike License or equivalent. Every chapter published in this book has been scrutinized by our experts. Their significance has been extensively debated. The topics covered herein carry significant information for a comprehensive understanding. They may even be implemented as practical applications or may be referred to as a beginning point for further studies.

We would like to thank the editorial team for lending their expertise to make the book truly unique. They have played a crucial role in the development of this book. Without their invaluable contributions this book wouldn't have been possible. They have made vital efforts to compile up to date information on the varied aspects of this subject to make this book a valuable addition to the collection of many professionals and students.

This book was conceptualized with the vision of imparting up-to-date and integrated information in this field. To ensure the same, a matchless editorial board was set up. Every individual on the board went through rigorous rounds of assessment to prove their worth. After which they invested a large part of their time researching and compiling the most relevant data for our readers.

The editorial board has been involved in producing this book since its inception. They have spent rigorous hours researching and exploring the diverse topics which have resulted in the successful publishing of this book. They have passed on their knowledge of decades through this book. To expedite this challenging task, the publisher supported the team at every step. A small team of assistant editors was also appointed to further simplify the editing procedure and attain best results for the readers.

Apart from the editorial board, the designing team has also invested a significant amount of their time in understanding the subject and creating the most relevant covers. They scrutinized every image to scout for the most suitable representation of the subject and create an appropriate cover for the book.

The publishing team has been an ardent support to the editorial, designing and production team. Their endless efforts to recruit the best for this project, has resulted in the accomplishment of this book. They are a veteran in the field of academics and their pool of knowledge is as vast as their experience in printing. Their expertise and guidance has proved useful at every step. Their uncompromising quality standards have made this book an exceptional effort. Their encouragement from time to time has been an inspiration for everyone.

The publisher and the editorial board hope that this book will prove to be a valuable piece of knowledge for students, practitioners and scholars across the globe.

INDEX

www.ingramcontent.com/pod-product-compliance
Lightning Source LLC
LaVergne TN
LVHW080627210926
848485LV00003B/221